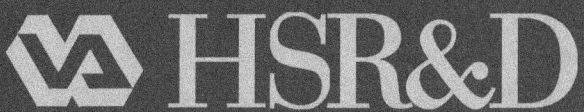

I0470863

A Systematic Evidence Review of Non-pharmacological Interventions for Behavioral Symptoms of Dementia

March 2011

Prepared for:
Department of Veterans Affairs
Veterans Health Administration
Health Services Research & Development Service
Washington, DC 20420

Prepared by:
Evidence-based Synthesis Program (ESP) Center
Portland VA Medical Center
Portland, OR
Devan Kansagara, MD, MCR, Director

Investigators:
Principal Investigator:
Maya E. O'Neil, PhD

Co-Investigators:
Michele Freeman, MPH
Vivian Christensen, PhD
Robin Telerant, MD
Ashlee Addleman, MPH
Devan Kansagara, MD, MCR

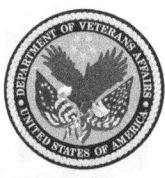

PREFACE

Health Services Research & Development Service's (HSR&D's) Evidence-based Synthesis Program (ESP) was established to provide timely and accurate syntheses of targeted healthcare topics of particular importance to Veterans Affairs (VA) managers and policymakers, as they work to improve the health and healthcare of Veterans. The ESP disseminates these reports throughout VA.

HSR&D provides funding for four ESP Centers and each Center has an active VA affiliation. The ESP Centers generate evidence syntheses on important clinical practice topics, and these reports help:

- develop clinical policies informed by evidence,
- guide the implementation of effective services to improve patient outcomes and to support VA clinical practice guidelines and performance measures, and
- set the direction for future research to address gaps in clinical knowledge.

In 2009, the ESP Coordinating Center was created to expand the capacity of HSR&D Central Office and the four ESP sites by developing and maintaining program processes. In addition, the Center established a Steering Committee comprised of HSR&D field-based investigators, VA Patient Care Services, Office of Quality and Performance, and Veterans Integrated Service Networks (VISN) Clinical Management Officers. The Steering Committee provides program oversight, guides strategic planning, coordinates dissemination activities, and develops collaborations with VA leadership to identify new ESP topics of importance to Veterans and the VA healthcare system.

Comments on this evidence report are welcome and can be sent to Nicole Floyd, ESP Coordinating Center Program Manager, at nicole.floyd@va.gov.

Recommended citation: O'Neil M, Freeman M, Christensen V, Telerant A, Addleman A, and Kansagara D. Non-pharmacological Interventions for Behavioral Symptoms of Dementia: A Systematic Review of the Evidence. VA-ESP Project #05-225; 2011

This report is based on research conducted by the Evidence-based Synthesis Program (ESP) Center located at the Portland VA Medical Center, Portland, OR funded by the Department of Veterans Affairs, Veterans Health Administration, Office of Research and Development, Health Services Research and Development. The findings and conclusions in this document are those of the author(s) who are responsible for its contents; the findings and conclusions do not necessarily represent the views of the Department of Veterans Affairs or the United States government. Therefore, no statement in this article should be construed as an official position of the Department of Veterans Affairs. No investigators have any affiliations or financial involvement (e.g., employment, consultancies, honoraria, stock ownership or options, expert testimony, grants or patents received or pending, or royalties) that conflict with material presented in the report.

TABLE OF CONTENTS

EXECUTIVE SUMMARY

BACKGROUND

In 2004, the Office of the Assistant Deputy Under Secretary for Health for Policy and Planning estimated that the total number of Veterans with dementia would be as high as 563,758 in FY 2010.[1] The VHA Office of Geriatrics and Extended Care (OGEC) in Patient Care Services has primary responsibility for coordination and direction of VHA dementia initiatives. OGEC convened an interdisciplinary Dementia Steering Committee (DSC) in December 2006, with the goal of making recommendations on comprehensive, coordinated care for Veterans with dementia.

The DSC requested VA HSR&D's Evidence-based Synthesis Program (ESP) to review evidence on selected topics, in order to assist with DSC planning efforts. This evidence review addresses the following questions:

Key Question #1. How do non-pharmacological treatments of behavioral symptoms compare in effectiveness with each other, with pharmacological approaches, and with no treatment?

Key Question #2. How do non-pharmacological treatments of behavioral symptoms compare in safety with each other, with pharmacological approaches, and with no treatment?

Key Question #3. How do non-pharmacological treatments of behavioral symptoms compare in cost with each other, with pharmacological approaches, and with no treatment?

METHODS

We conducted searches for systematic reviews of non-pharmacological interventions for dementia in MEDLINE (PubMed), using the following search terms: ("dementia"[MeSH Terms] OR "dementia"[All Fields]) AND systematic[sb]. We also searched in the Cochrane Database of Systematic Reviews and the Cochrane Database of Reviews of Effects (OVID) from database inception through July 2009, using the term dementia.mp. We obtained additional articles from reference lists of pertinent studies. We conducted a separate search for primary studies of animal-assisted therapies because there were no existing systematic reviews on this topic. Additional primary studies were suggested for inclusion by reviewers based on recency and relevance to the field. We summarized the findings of good quality systematic reviews of the primary literature on the various non-pharmacological interventions.

RESULTS

We identified 21 good quality systematic reviews that each examined a single non-pharmacological intervention, and seven good quality systematic reviews that reviewed a variety of interventions. Cognitive/emotion-oriented interventions were reviewed in 10 reports, sensory stimulation interventions in 12 reports, and behavior management techniques in 3 reports. We also added two primary studies related to behavior management techniques identified by our expert panel as neither of these more recent primary articles were included in previous systematic reviews. Three reports reviewed exercise. The search for primary studies of animal-assisted therapies yielded nine prospective studies. Five reports reviewed a variety of interventions for wandering, and one report reviewed various interventions for agitation. Additionally, we added one primary study related to agitation identified by our expert panel as this recent study was not included in the previous systematic reviews. The findings for specific intervention types are summarized below.

Summary of Findings

Key Question #1. How do non-pharmacological treatments of behavioral symptoms compare in effectiveness with each other, with pharmacological approaches, and with no treatment?

Cognitive/Emotion-oriented Interventions

Reminiscence Therapy: Reminiscence therapy involves the discussion of past activities, events, and experiences with another person or a group of people. Two previous systematic reviews identified seven small randomized control trials (RCTs) of reminiscence therapy. This limited body of evidence does not support the use of reminiscence therapy for the treatment of behavioral symptoms of dementia.

Simulated Presence Therapy (SPT): SPT involves the use of audiotapes made by family members containing a scripted conversation about cherished memories about the patient's life. Overall, well-conducted studies are lacking, the evidence that SPT reduces behavioral symptoms of dementia is inconsistent, and SPT may have adverse effects in some patients.

Validation Therapy: Validation therapy is intended to give the individual an opportunity to resolve unfinished conflicts by encouraging and validating expressions of feeling. Four systematic reviews examined the effects of validation therapy in three RCTs as well as other study designs, and found mixed effects. Overall, there is insufficient evidence to draw conclusions about the efficacy of validation therapy for behavioral symptoms, depression, and emotional state associated with dementia.

Sensory Stimulation Interventions

Acupuncture: Acupuncture is an ancient Chinese treatment that has been used for over 3,000 years. One systematic review found no rigorously conducted RCTs. There is no good quality evidence indicating benefit or harm of acupuncture for the treatment of behavioral symptoms for dementia.

Aromatherapy: Aromatherapy consists of the use of fragrant oils from plants, and has been used to promote sleep and reduce behavioral symptoms in individuals with dementia. Overall, there is insufficient evidence that aromatherapy may be an effective treatment for agitation and other behavioral symptoms.

Light Therapy: Light stimulation aims to improve the circadian disturbances in the sleep-wake cycles experienced by individuals with dementia. Two systematic reviews identified six studies, including two RCTs. Although some studies found beneficial effects of bright light therapy on agitation and nocturnal restlessness, studies were generally limited by small sample size and poor quality. The limited body of evidence is insufficient to draw definitive conclusions about the effects of bright light therapy in managing sleep, behavior, or mood disturbances associated with dementia.

Massage and Touch: Massage and touch therapies aim to reduce depression, anxiety, and other behavioral symptoms of dementia. A systematic review identified two small RCTs that reported increased calorie and protein intake in a study that compared touch combined with verbal encouragement during meals to verbal encouragement alone, and reduced agitation in a study that compared hand massage with calming music and with no treatment. This limited body of evidence suggests that, compared with no treatment, hand massage and touch therapy may have beneficial effects.

Music Therapy: Individuals with dementia may retain the ability to sing old songs, and musical abilities appear to be preserved in some individuals despite aphasia and memory loss. Music interventions range from activities administered by a professional music therapist to the presentation of recorded music by caregivers to patients in an individual or group setting. We identified four systematic reviews that examined a variety of study designs. Three RCTs reported reduced aggression, agitation, and wandering while listening to music; and other studies found similar reductions in behavioral symptoms, although there was no evidence of long-term effects. All studies were limited by methodological issues. Overall, well-conducted studies are lacking, but music interventions have potential for reducing agitation in patients with dementia in the short term.

Snoezelen Multisensory Stimulation Therapy: Multisensory stimulation (MSS), otherwise known as Snoezelen therapy, combines the therapeutic use of light, tactile surfaces, music, and aroma. MSS is based on the premise that neuropsychiatric symptoms may result from periods of sensory deprivation. There were six RCTs identified among four systematic reviews. Although the evidence did not consistently demonstrate a durable effect of MSS therapy on behavioral symptoms, preliminary findings of short-term benefits and the reported pleasantness of the treatment suggest that future research is warranted.

Transcutaneous Electrical Nerve Stimulation (TENS): TENS is a non-invasive analgesic technique that is most often used for pain control and occasionally for neurological and psychiatric conditions, such as drug/alcohol dependency, headaches, and depression. A systematic review combined data from three RCTs in individuals with dementia and found no significant effects on sleep disturbances or behavioral symptoms, evaluated immediately after treatment or at six-week follow-up. Although some short-lived improvements in neuropsychological symptoms of dementia have been observed with TENS, definite conclusions on the possible benefits of this intervention cannot be made.

Behavior Management Techniques

Behavior management techniques include a wide variety of behavioral interventions such as functional analysis of specific behaviors, token economies, habit training, progressive muscle relaxation, communication training, behavioral or cognitive-behavioral therapy, and various types of individualized behavioral reinforcement strategies. Findings from three systematic reviews including seven RCTs and two additional more recent trials provide some support for behavior management techniques as effective interventions for behavioral symptoms of dementia. However, mixed study results, the variety of specific interventions across studies, and methodological concerns in many studies suggest that additional research in this area replicating results is warranted.

Other Psychosocial Interventions

Animal-assisted Therapy: There were no RCTs evaluating the effectiveness or harm of pet therapy. Nine non-randomized studies demonstrated decreases in agitated and disrupted behaviors, increases in social and verbal interactions, decreases in passivity, and increases in nutritional intake. The findings suggest that pet therapy has potential for benefit, but more rigorous studies are needed to establish benefit, harms, and feasibility for implementation in VA settings.

Exercise: Three systematic reviews of 59 studies showed inconsistent effects of exercise interventions on behavioral symptoms and functional status. Variations in intensity of exercise intervention, severity of dementia at baseline, and outcome measures make it difficult to draw a firm conclusion. Many of the included studies were small and did not use rigorous methodology. The most consistent evidence showed that exercise did increase sleep duration and decrease nighttime awakenings. While the impact of improved sleep on distal health outcomes remains uncertain, there may be an additional benefit to caregivers who are disproportionally affected by dysfunctional sleep.

Various Interventions Targeting a Specific Behavioral Symptom

Wandering: A variety of interventions for wandering were examined in four systematic reviews. There were no RCTs on the effects of subjective visual barriers, such as mirrors, floor grids, camouflage of doors or doorknobs, and concealment of view through door windows. Two RCTs determined that exercise and walking therapies had no impact on wandering. No evidence is available on the effects of wander gardens. Tracking devices, motion detection devices, and home alarms were generally effective in detecting wandering and locating lost patients in non-randomized studies. Evidence about the effects of sensory stimulation therapies, such as MSS, aromatherapy, and music on wandering, is scant and inconclusive.

Agitation: A systematic review of agitation identified 14 RCTs of a variety of interventions. Three studies of sensory interventions (aromatherapy, thermal bath, calming music, and hand massage) showed a statistically significant decrease in agitation when combined in meta-analysis, but there was substantial variability in the type of intervention, duration of exposure, and outcomes measured. Other interventions including social contact, environmental modification, caregiver training, and behavior therapy showed no effects on agitation. One recently conducted primary study suggested to us by reviewers provided preliminary support for the effectiveness of systematic individualized intervention in decreasing agitation, though a lack of assessor blinding to condition limits the validity of these findings.

Inappropriate Sexual Behavior: There were no systematic reviews that examined the topic of inappropriate sexual behavior among individuals with dementia. Currently, the effectiveness of non-pharmacological treatments for inappropriate sexual behavior is unknown.

Comparative effectiveness among non-pharmacological interventions and between pharmacological and non-pharmacological approaches

None of the systematic reviews captured in our search identified any head-to-head trials that directly compared effectiveness among different non-pharmacological interventions, or between non-pharmacological and pharmacological treatments.

Key Question #2. How do non-pharmacological treatments of behavioral symptoms compare in safety with each other, with pharmacological approaches, and with no treatment?

Cognitive/Emotion-oriented Interventions: One study found that simulated presence therapy increased agitation and disruptive behaviors in some patients. Reality orientation has been observed by caregivers to increase distress, fear, and agitation in individuals with later stages of dementia.

Sensory Stimulation Interventions: For some individuals, the increased stimulation from sensory stimulation therapies such as music therapy and massage/touch therapy may cause increased agitation and aggression. Consideration of the individual preferences in the use of these treatments should be emphasized.

Behavior Management Techniques: None of the systematic reviews nor the primary studies reviewed documented any patient harm or safety concerns resulting from the use of behavior management techniques.

Animal-assisted Therapy: The American Veterinary Medical Association guidelines describe potential physical and emotional harms associated with animal-assisted therapy, but the actual incidence of harms has not been well-studied. Theoretical harms include human injury, zoonotic disease, allergic reactions, and the risk of grief reaction if an animal dies.

Exercise: Potential harms of exercise programs include the increased risk of falls or physical injuries, but risks associated with exercise have not been well studied.

Comparative Safety among Non-pharmacological Interventions and between Pharmacological and Non-pharmacological Approaches

None of the systematic reviews captured in our search identified any head-to-head trials that directly compared safety among different non-pharmacological interventions, or between non-pharmacological and pharmacological treatments.

Key Question #3: How do non-pharmacological treatments of behavioral symptoms compare in cost with each other, with pharmacological approaches, and with no treatment?

None of the systematic reviews or primary articles we retrieved identified direct evidence on the cost-effectiveness of specific interventions. The costs associated with the use of GPS tracking devices and other monitoring systems are high, but the potential increases in patient safety and caregiver peace of mind associated with the use of these devices are notable. The training and veterinary care required for preparing and maintaining a live animal for animal-assisted therapy are costly. Some forms of animal-assisted therapy such as the placement of aquariums in dining areas may be less expensive than more individualized approaches. Behavior management techniques can include a variety of individualized interventions, and therefore expense for these techniques can vary greatly across individuals and settings. Further studies are needed to determine the cost-benefits, harms, and feasibility of these and other non-pharmacological interventions.

EVIDENCE REPORT

INTRODUCTION

BACKGROUND

In 2004, the Office of the Assistant Deputy Under Secretary for Health for Policy and Planning estimated that the total number of Veterans with dementia would be as high as 563,758 in FY 2010.[1] The behavioral symptoms that are associated with dementia, such as agitation/aggression, wandering, and sleep disturbances, are associated with increased caregiver burden, decreased quality of life for the patient, and increased healthcare costs.[2,3] It is estimated that behavioral symptoms occur in as many as 90 percent of people with Alzheimer's disease (AD).[4] Moreover, it is the behavioral symptoms that are most often cited by caregivers as the reason for the placement of individuals with dementia into residential care.[5]

Psychotropic medications are commonly used to reduce the frequency and severity of the behavioral symptoms of dementia. There is little evidence, however, that such interventions are effective,[3,6] and their potential side effects are frequent and often hazardous.[5,6] It has been reported that the use of atypical and typical antipsychotic medication is associated with the increased risk of death.[6,7]

Because of the limited benefits and the potential harms associated with psychotropic medications, non-pharmacological interventions for the behavioral symptoms associated with dementia may be an attractive alternative to pharmacological treatment. The purpose of this report is to review systematically the evidence on non-pharmacological treatments for behavioral symptoms of dementia.

METHODS

TOPIC DEVELOPMENT

The review was requested by the VHA Dementia Steering Committee (DSC) and commissioned by the Department of Veterans Affairs' Evidence-based Synthesis Program. The DSC served as the technical expert panel for guiding topic development and reviewing drafts of the report. The objective of this report is to review the evidence that addresses the following questions:

Key Question #1. How do non-pharmacological treatments of behavioral symptoms compare in effectiveness with each other, with pharmacological approaches, and with no treatment?

Key Question #2. How do non-pharmacological treatments of behavioral symptoms compare in safety with each other, with pharmacological approaches, and with no treatment?

Key Question #3. How do non-pharmacological treatments of behavioral symptoms compare in cost with each other, with pharmacological approaches, and with no treatment?

Population: Adults with mild, moderate, or severe dementia.

Behavioral symptoms: Apathy, agitation, disruptive vocalizations, aggression, disturbed sleep, wandering, impulsivity, disinhibition, depression, inappropriate sexual behavior, chronic/intermittent hallucinations and delusions.

Interventions: Non-pharmacological treatments include cognitive/emotion-oriented interventions (e.g., reminiscence therapy, simulated presence therapy, and validation therapy), sensory stimulation interventions (e.g., acupuncture, aromatherapy, light therapy, massage/touch therapy, music therapy, Snoezelen multisensory stimulation, and Transcutaneous Electrical Nerve Stimulation (TENS)), behavior management techniques, other psychosocial interventions (e.g., animal-assisted therapy and exercise), and various interventions targeting a specific behavioral symptom (e.g., wandering, agitation, and inappropriate sexual behavior).

Comparators: Routine care; medical (e.g., ECT)/pharmacological treatment (e.g., typical and atypical antipsychotics, benzodiazepines and their pharmacological relatives, cholinesterase inhibitors, mood stabilizers, anti-depressants, N-Methyl-D-aspartic acid receptor antagonists); other non-pharmacological treatment; or no treatment.

Outcomes: Use of psychotropic drugs; cognition; mood, behavioral symptoms; social function, or physical function; hospitalizations, institutionalizations, or healthcare visits including ER visits; accidents, such as accidental falls or automobile crashes; mortality; health-related quality of life; and satisfaction with healthcare.

Setting: All outpatient care settings including home-based care and ambulatory care, and extended-care facility settings. Treatments for acute psychotic episodes are excluded.

SEARCH STRATEGY

We conducted searches for systematic reviews of non-pharmacological interventions for dementia in MEDLINE (PubMed), the Cochrane Database of Systematic Reviews, the Cochrane

Database of Reviews of Effects (OVID), and PsycInfo from database inception through September 2009 (Appendix A). We obtained additional articles from reference lists of pertinent studies. Additional articles were obtained through reviewer feedback following review of the initial draft of this report. All citations were imported into an electronic database (EndNote X2).

Because the initial search identified no systematic reviews on animal-assisted therapy, we proceeded to conduct a search for primary studies (Appendix B).

STUDY SELECTION AND QUALITY ASSESSMENT

We included good quality systematic reviews of non-pharmacological interventions in individuals with dementia, but excluded interventions that targeted primarily caregiver outcomes as we had conducted a separate review of this topic.[8] Two reviewers assessed the titles and abstracts identified by the literature search for relevance to the key questions. Potentially relevant full-text articles were retrieved for further review. Each article was reviewed using the eligibility criteria for systematic reviews shown in Appendix C. The quality rating of systematic reviews (see criteria, Appendix D) is based on the comprehensiveness and reproducibility of the search strategy, the use of standard methods to appraise the validity of included studies, and the absence of apparent bias in drawing conclusions. Because technological interventions such as GPS tracking devices are recent innovations and not widely studied, we allowed inclusion of fair quality reviews of these technologies.

We conducted a search for primary studies of the effects of animal-assisted therapy on behavioral symptoms (inclusion criteria Appendix E), as no systematic reviews were available. We did not limit by study design, other than excluding case series and case reports, and rather than report a summary quality score, we noted limitations of individual studies.

DATA SYNTHESIS

We organized the literature into the following categories:

- Cognitive/emotion-oriented interventions
  - Reminiscence therapy
  - Simulated presence therapy
  - Validation therapy
- Sensory stimulation interventions
  - Acupuncture
  - Aromatherapy
  - Light therapy
  - Massage/touch
  - Music therapy
  - Snoezelen multisensory stimulation
  - TENS
- Behavior management techniques (BMT)
- Other psychosocial interventions
  - Animal-assisted therapy
  - Exercise

- Various interventions targeting a specific behavioral symptom
  - Wandering
  - Agitation

We compiled a qualitative synthesis of the evidence on specific forms of therapy, and on various therapies targeting wandering and wandering behaviors. Given the breadth and complexity of studies on behavior management techniques, as well as stakeholder interest, we examined randomized controlled trials (RCTs) with sample size > 30 that were identified in previous systematic reviews, and additional studies of behavior management techniques that were referred to us by peer reviewers. Additionally, based on reviewer feedback, we included one primary study on agitation which was not captured in the review due to its recency.

We assessed the overall quality of evidence for outcomes using a method developed by the GRADE Working Group.[9] The GRADE method considers the consistency, coherence, and applicability of a body of evidence, as well as the internal validity of individual studies to classify the grade of evidence across outcomes. The grade of evidence is rated as high, moderate, low, or very low, based on the confidence in the estimate of effect and the likelihood that future research would have an important impact on the certainty, magnitude, or direction of the estimate.

A list of abbreviations and their definitions is provided in Appendix F.

PEER REVIEW

A draft version of this report was sent to the technical advisory panel and additional peer reviewers. Their comments and our responses are included in Appendix G.

RESULTS

LITERATURE SEARCH

The search for systematic reviews yielded 556 citations, of which 114 were retained. An additional six articles were suggested by reviewers following initial draft review, resulting in a total of 120 articles for full-text review (Figure 1). Of these, we included 28 systematic reviews that met our quality criteria (Appendix D) and three primary studies not cited in previous systematic reviews. We additionally included a systematic review that did not fully meet our quality criteria, but contributed relevant information about recently developed technology-based interventions.

The search for primary studies of animal-assisted therapies yielded 380 abstracts, of which 65 were retrieved for full-text review (Figure 2). Nine studies provided data that addressed the key questions in this review.

Non-pharmacological Interventions for Behavioral Symptoms of Dementia

Figure 1. Literature flow for systematic reviews

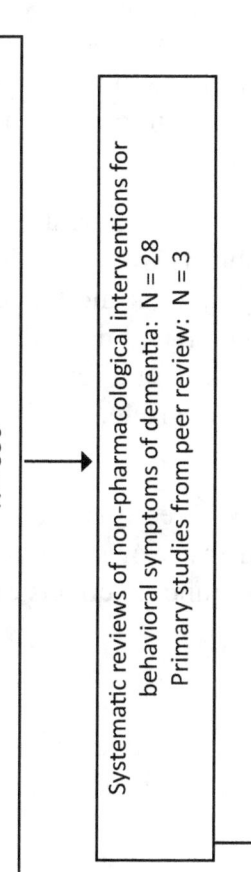

Figure 2. Literature flow for primary studies of animal-assisted therapy

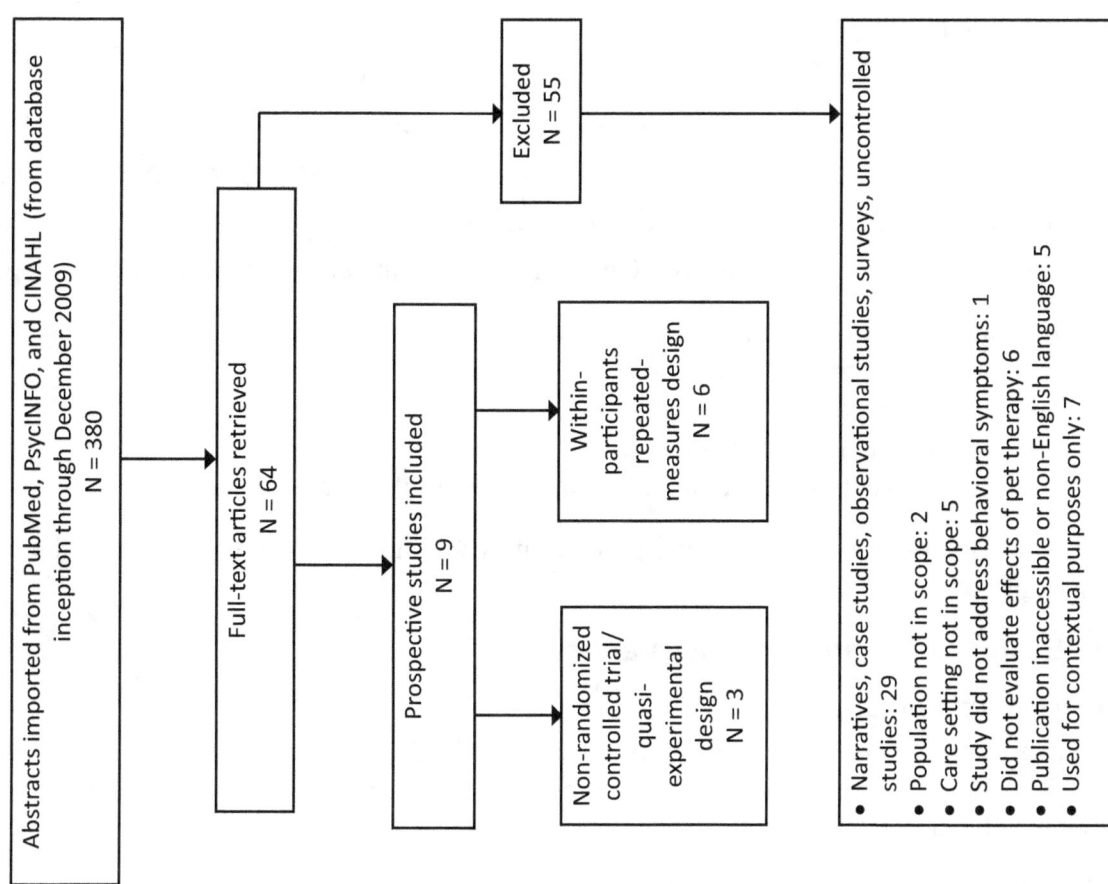

KEY QUESTION #1. How do non-pharmacological treatments of behavioral symptoms compare in effectiveness with each other, with pharmacological approaches, and with no treatment?

The review of evidence addressing Key Question #1 is organized into the following categories:

- Cognitive/emotion-oriented interventions
- Sensory stimulation interventions
- Behavior management techniques
- Other psychosocial interventions
- Various interventions targeting a specific behavioral symptom

The organization of evidence on specific interventions within each category follows the order shown in Figure 1.

Cognitive/Emotion-oriented Interventions

Reminiscence Therapy

Summary: With the exception of one small trial (N=17) that showed a benefit on mood, this limited body of evidence of small trials does not support the use of reminiscence therapy for the treatment of behavioral symptoms of dementia.

Details: Reminiscence therapy involves the discussion of past activities, events and experiences with another person or group of people. Reminiscence therapy uses materials such as old newspapers, photographs, household and other familiar items from the past to stimulate memories and enable people to share and value their experiences.[10, 11] General reminiscence in a group context aims to enhance interaction, whereas life review usually involves individual sessions in which the person is guided chronologically through life experiences and encouraged to evaluate them. Studies have suggested that reminiscence work assists in reducing depression in older people, and both of these approaches might plausibly have an impact on mood and well-being.[10]

We found one systematic review that focused on reminiscence therapy as a treatment for dementia.[10] Four RCTs that included a combined total of 144 subjects were included in the findings of this review. Three of the RCTs assessed behavioral symptoms and found no effect of reminiscence therapy on these symptoms. One RCT (N=17) compared the effects of 12 individual weekly sessions of reminiscence therapy with no treatment, and found statistically significant improvements in depression at six weeks in the treatment group, but found no differences in other behavioral symptoms between groups.[10]

A systematic review examining a variety of interventions included three small RCTs (combined N=38) of reminiscence therapy, and found no clear benefit.[11] Other reviews that examined reminiscence therapy in addition to other interventions similarly found no effects of reminiscence therapy on behavioral symptoms.[4, 12]

Simulated Presence Therapy (SPT)

Summary: The findings of the included studies are mixed, and well-conducted studies are lacking. This body of research did not find consistent evidence that SPT reduces behavioral symptoms of dementia. In addition, there is some indication that SPT may worsen behavioral symptoms of dementia in some individuals.

Details: Simulated presence therapy (SPT) involves the use of audiotapes made by family members containing scripted "telephone conversations" about cherished memories from earlier life, in an effort to tap remote memory, improve behavioral symptoms, and enhance quality of life among persons with dementia.[3, 13]

Our search identified one systematic review that focused on SPT for the treatment of behavioral symptoms of dementia.[3] A meta-analysis found a statistically significant effect of SPT on disruptive, agitated, or depressed behaviors from pre- to post-intervention, but this analysis was based on three small quasi-experimental studies (ranging from six to nine subjects in each) and one small RCT (N=30). Furthermore, there was significant statistical heterogeneity between studies and substantial variation in the research designs used, the measures used to assess challenging behavior, and the administration of SPT. The review identified three additional studies that could not be combined in the meta-analysis; of these, two studies found that SPT was effective in reducing challenging behaviors, and the third found no overall benefit and that the response to SPT may differ among individuals. Furthermore, three studies identified in the review reported that SPT actually increased agitation or disruptive behaviors in some participants. The authors of the review noted the importance of assessing participants' suitability for emotion-oriented approaches and monitoring their responses closely.[3]

A review of multiple interventions included one non-randomized controlled study of SPT vs. recorded readings from a newspaper and found no statistically significant differences in monitored behaviors.[12]

Validation Therapy

Summary: The findings are mixed, and the evidence is insufficient to draw conclusions about the efficacy of the treatment of validation therapy for dementia.

Details: Validation therapy is based on the general principle of validation, the acceptance of the reality and personal truth of another's experience, and incorporates a range of specific techniques.[14] Validation therapy is intended to give the individual an opportunity to resolve unfinished conflicts by encouraging and validating expression of feelings.[11]

One systematic review focused on validation therapy for the treatment of dementia.[14] The review included three RCTs with a combined total of 146 subjects. Comparison groups in the studies included usual care, social contact (activities such as music, art, literature, dance, and games), and reality orientation. One study compared the effects of validation therapy, reality orientation, and usual care on behavioral symptoms among 31 nursing home residents. Participants in the treatment group received 30-minute validation sessions, five days a week, for six weeks. At the end of the treatment period, the study found a significant difference in Behavior Assessment Tool (BAT) scores in favor of validation therapy compared to usual care, but there were no significant differences between validation therapy and reality orientation therapy. The second study compared usual care to validation therapy (30-minute sessions, four days per week for 52 weeks) given to 27 residents of a large VA Medical Center (VAMC). The study found no significant differences in behavior after nine months of therapy. In a study of 88 patients from four nursing homes, a beneficial effect on depression was observed at 12 months in favor of validation therapy compared with social contact, but there was no difference compared to usual care.

Three additional systematic reviews that examined validation therapy in addition to other forms of therapy found no statistically significant findings in favor of validation therapy for reducing behavioral symptoms of dementia.[4, 11, 12]

Sensory Stimulation Interventions

Acupuncture

Summary: There are currently no good quality trials evaluating acupuncture for the treatment of behavioral symptoms associated with dementia.

Details: Acupuncture is an ancient Chinese method which has been used for both the prevention and treatment of diseases for over 3,000 years.[15] One systematic review evaluated acupuncture in patients with vascular dementia.[15] The review found 17 RCTs, but found them all to be ineligible for the following reasons: 1) the control group received some form of Western medicine in six studies; 2) there was inadequate randomization in four studies; 3) acupuncture was used in conjunction with another therapy and the effects of acupuncture could not be evaluated separately in six studies; and 4) insufficient information was available for one study. Because none of the identified RCTs met inclusion criteria for this review, the effectiveness and safety of acupuncture could not be analyzed. The authors of the review emphasized the need for randomized placebo-controlled trials of acupuncture.[15]

Aromatherapy

Summary: There is limited evidence that aromatherapy may be an effective treatment for the behavioral symptom of agitation.

Details: Aromatherapy consists of the use of fragrant oils from plants. Aromatherapy has been used in attempts to reduce behavioral symptoms, to promote sleep, and to stimulate motivational behavior in people with dementia.[16] Much of the literature on aromatherapy comes from qualitative research and small scale non-randomized trials.[16]

One systematic review focused solely on aromatherapy, but only one RCT met its inclusion criteria.[16] This clustered RCT included 72 participants with severe dementia in eight nursing homes. The four-week study examined the effects of topical Melissa oil, and sunflower oil was used at control nursing homes. Though the study found a significant decrease in measures of agitation and neuropsychiatric symptoms, there was no significant decrease in aggression, and important differences among participants such as medication use were not accounted for.

A study cited in another systematic review[13] similarly found that aromatherapy was associated with decreased agitation among dementia patients. In this study of 15 individuals, two percent lavender oil or water vapor was sprayed in a communal area of a dementia ward for two hours a day, on alternating days for 10 sessions. Agitation was assessed during the last hour of each session using the Pittsburgh Agitation Scale, by an observer who wore a nose clip in an effort to be blinded to the intervention. Median behavior scores were 20 percent lower while exposed to lavender compared to water vapor, and the difference was statistically significant (p= 0.016).[13]

Light Therapy

Summary: There is insufficient evidence to draw any conclusions about the effectiveness of bright light therapy in managing sleep, behavior, or mood disturbances associated with dementia.

Details: Rest-activity and sleep-wake cycles are controlled by the endogenous circadian rhythm generated by the suprachiasmatic nuclei (SCN) of the hypothalamus. Degenerative changes in the SCN appear to be a biological basis of circadian disturbances in people with dementia. In addition to the internal regulatory loss, elderly people (especially those with dementia) experience a reduction in sensory input because they are visually less sensitive to light and have less exposure to bright environmental light. Evidence suggests that circadian disturbances may be reversed by stimulation of the SCN by light.[17]

One Cochrane review examined RCTs of the effects of light therapy on sleep, behavior, and mood disturbances among patients with dementia in long-term care facilities.[17] Only two studies met methodological and design criteria for inclusion in the review. One small RCT compared dawn-dusk simulation (maximum 400 lux) to dim red light (<5 lux) for three weeks among 13 nursing home residents. There were no significant differences in any outcome: nocturnal sleep duration, night-time activity, sleep latency (defined as the amount of time between reclining in bed and the onset of sleep), agitation (Neuropsychiatric Inventory; NPI), and depression (Geriatric Depression Scale; GDS) measured at the end of light therapy and three weeks post-treatment.

Another RCT randomly assigned 92 nursing home residents with severe Alzheimer's disease to receive morning bright light, evening bright light, or morning dim red light for 10 days. The study found no differences between groups in sleep duration or agitation at the end of therapy and at five days post-treatment.

An older systematic review included four studies of bright light therapy, three of which reported beneficial effects on agitation and nocturnal restlessness during bright light treatment (1500 – 2500 lux).[5] The studies were limited by small sample size (N ≤ 24), and three of the studies had samples of 10 subjects or fewer.

Massage and Touch Therapy

Summary: Though the true effect of massage and touch on behavioral symptoms is uncertain, this very small body of evidence preliminarily suggests that hand massage and touch may be a viable treatment option, especially given the ease of implementation and minimal training involved.

Details: Massage and touch are among the interventions used in dementia care with the aim of reducing depression, anxiety, aggression and other related psychological and behavioral manifestations.[18] Expressive touch such as patting or holding a client's hand involves emotional intent, for example, to calm a patient or to show concern, as opposed to instrumental/task-associated touch within nursing care.[19]

A 2005 review focused on RCTs of massage and touch therapies for dementia.[18] Eligibility criteria required that studies used a RCT design, employed blinding of outcome assessors, and measured changes in agitated behavior. Of 34 references identified by the search, only two small RCTs met these criteria. One RCT of 42 institutionalized patients with organic brain syndrome compared verbal encouragement with touch to verbal encouragement alone during meals, and found that touch therapy was associated with a significant increase in mean calorie and protein intake. The second RCT assessed the effect of hand massage vs. calming music, and simultaneous hand massage and calming music vs. no intervention. Sixty-eight participants were randomly assigned to one of four groups. Interventions consisted of a single 10-minute treatment. Researchers found a greater decrease in agitated behavior (CMAI score) compared with baseline during treatment, immediately after treatment, and one hour after treatment among the groups receiving hand massage compared to the group receiving no treatment. Findings were similar for hand massage, calming music, or both.

Another systematic review that examined touch interventions among other treatments for dementia identified a small RCT that found that an expressive touch intervention that involved 5.5 minutes a day of touching, including 2.5 minutes a day of gentle massage and 3 minutes a day of intermittent touching with someone talking, over a 10-day period decreased disturbed behavior from baseline immediately and for 5 days after the intervention.[11]

Music Therapy

Summary: Music interventions have potential for reducing agitation in persons with dementia in the short-term. Well-conducted studies are lacking, and trials with adequate sample size and rigorous methodology are needed. Some interventions such as listening to recorded music during mealtimes are simple and low-cost, and they may be feasible in VA settings. The feasibility and cost-effectiveness of more resource-intensive interventions, such as individual patient interactions with a professional music therapist, need to be evaluated.

Details: People with dementia may retain the ability to sing old songs,[20, 21] and musical abilities appear to be preserved in individuals with dementia who were musicians[22] despite aphasia and memory loss. Information presented in a song context appears to enhance retention and recall of information, and structured music activities can promote interaction and communication. Music therapy can, therefore, potentially enhance cognitive skills as well as social/emotional skills, and may also serve as an alternative to medication for managing behavioral symptoms of AD.[23] There is a wide range of music interventions for older people with dementia, including listening to different types of music, instrument playing, or group exercise while listening to music. The range of music interventions includes activities administered by a professional music therapist, as well as the presentation of recorded music by a variety of caregivers, to patients privately or in a group setting.

The literature search for music and music therapy interventions for behavioral symptoms identified 18 reviews that included a total of 104 primary studies. Among these reviews, we selected four systematic reviews[11, 24-26] based on quality, recency, and relevance. The most rigorous systematic review was a Cochrane review[24] that conducted a literature search through September 2005, and included three RCTs.[27-29] Three other systematic reviews included a wider range of study designs not limited to RCTs.[11, 25, 26]

The Cochrane review[24] determined that trials were poor in quality, citing inadequate reporting of methods of randomization and blinding, as well as inappropriate methods of data analysis in two of the studies.[27, 28] Reviewers concluded that no study presented any quantitative results in sufficient detail to justify the original investigators' conclusions that music listening was more effective than control on behavioral symptoms.[24] In one study, when bathing was accompanied by listening to preferred music (as compared with no music), residents demonstrated significantly less aggressive behaviors.[27] Gerdner (2000) reports that agitation was significantly less frequent during and after music therapy when each patient listened to his or her preferred music compared with standard classical music.[28] Groene (1993) reported that the amount of time a wandering subject remained seated or in close proximity to the session area was longer for music sessions than for reading sessions.[29]

Systematic reviews that included a wider range of study designs consistently concluded that music therapy decreases agitation in the short-term, although there was no evidence of long-term effects. One systematic review examined 20 studies published through 2000,[26] and another included 24 music interventions (including 14 of the same studies) published through 2003.[11] A systematic review of eight studies that specifically examined the use of preferred or individualized music found reductions in agitated behaviors that were statistically significant in all but one study.[25]

Methodological limitations in the music intervention studies include lack of randomization, observational methods and sampling techniques, problems with internal validity, and confounding due to the possible effects of the music intervention on staff. Some studies employed momentary time sampling techniques, where the observer records whether or not the behavior is occurring at the end of a pre-specified time period. This sampling method may tend to overestimate continuous behaviors and underestimate discrete episodes of behavior. Internal validity was questionable in two studies in which some participants were transferred to "geri-chairs" that prevent the patient from leaving the chair due to a fixed tray across the chair arms. A reduction in agitation behaviors in these studies was attributed to the effects of music, despite the fact that the use of these chairs would directly affect pacing behaviors.[26] In another study, the effects of the music intervention on staff behavior was an unexpected confounder.[30] This study compared the use of taped music to no music during mealtimes, and it measured the amount of food eaten by participants. The participants' consumption of food increased during the music conditions, but the staff served more food during the music conditions as well. The effect of music on increasing food intake could not be clearly separated from the fact that the patients had received more food on their plates.

Snoezelen Multisensory Stimulation Therapy

Summary: There is no consistent evidence demonstrating a durable effect of multisensory stimulation (MSS) therapy on behavioral symptoms of dementia. Preliminary findings of short-term benefits and the reported pleasantness of the treatment of MSS, however, suggest that future research may be warranted.

Details: MSS, otherwise known as Snoezelen therapy, is based on the premise that neuropsychiatric symptoms may result from periods of sensory deprivation.[11, 31] MSS uses multiple stimuli during a treatment session aimed at stimulating the primary senses of sight, hearing, touch, taste and smell. MSS combines the use of such treatments as lights, tactile surfaces, music, and aroma.[31] Interventions generally occur in specially designed rooms with a variety of sensory based materials. A typical MSS room provides taped music, aroma, bubble tubes, fiber optic sprays and moving shapes projected across walls.[12] MSS has become a popular intervention for behavioral symptoms in persons with dementia, but the application of MSS varies in form, procedures, and in frequency of treatment.[31]

One systematic review included two RCTs in which MSS was used for a total of 246 individuals with dementia aged 60 and older.[31] The first study compared eight 30-minute MSS sessions to activity sessions that were based on individual subjects' preferences and abilities, but with no obvious sensory inputs. No significant effects on mood were found either immediately after intervention or at one-month post-follow-up. The second study compared a 24-hour exposure to MSS with usual care. Although patients appeared to find MSS enjoyable, the study found no long-term significant effects on behavior or mood.

Other systematic reviews[11, 12, 32] identified four additional RCTs and reported mixed results. One study administered MSS in specially designed rooms in 30- to 60-minute sessions and found that during the four-week treatment period, disruptive behavior outside the treatment setting briefly improved but did not last once the treatment had stopped. Two studies conducted MSS sessions for 30 to 60 minutes for three consecutive days and found that subjects were less apathetic when remaining in a multisensory stimulation room compared with remaining in the living room or receiving activity therapy. Lastly, one small (N=20) repeated-measures study set in a day-care center and mental health nursing home exposed patients to three 40-minute sessions of either MSS or reminiscence therapy and found no significant differences in behavior symptoms during or after treatment.

Transcutaneous Electrical Nerve Stimulation (TENS)

Summary: Although some short-lived improvements in neuropsychological symptoms of dementia have been observed with TENS, definite conclusions on the possible benefits of this intervention cannot be made.

Details: TENS is a simple, non-invasive analgesic technique that is most often used for pain control and occasionally for neurological and psychiatric conditions such as drug/alcohol dependency, headaches, and depression.[33, 34] TENS is the application of an electrical current through electrodes attached to the skin. Short, pulsed electrical currents are generated by a portable pulse generator and delivered across the intact surface of the skin through conditioning pads called electrodes.[33] By carefully adjusting the intensity and duration of the pulses, a mild tingling sensation without pain or muscle contraction, or a stronger sensation involving muscle contraction, can be produced.[34] Few known side effects exist and there are no known drug interactions.[33] Although TENS is not routinely used for treatment of dementia, several studies in the Netherlands and one study in Japan suggest that TENS applied to the back or head may improve cognition, behavior, and sleep disorders in patients with Alzheimer's disease or multi-infarct dementia.[34]

We identified one systematic review of the effectiveness of TENS in the treatment of dementia.[34] The review reported that TENS produced a statistically significant improvement directly after treatment in delayed recall of eight words in one trial, face recognition in two trials and motivation in one trial, but there were no significant effects of TENS treatment on sleep disorders or behavior disorders evaluated immediately after treatment or at six-week post-treatment. Of nine RCTs identified, only three of the studies provided sufficient data to be combined in a pooled analysis, for a combined total of 63 subjects. Two of these studies were conducted in the Netherlands, and one was conducted in Japan. In one study, TENS was provided for 30 minutes per day, five days per week for six weeks; in another study, TENS was applied for six hours per day; in the Japanese study, TENS was applied for 20 minutes daily for two weeks. In each study, a placebo treatment was delivered using electrodes that were disconnected from the device. The only adverse effects mentioned were from the Japanese study in which one patient to whom cranial electrical stimulation was applied complained of a dull pain in the head with active treatment. None of the other studies mentioned adverse effects, although it is unclear if adverse events were monitored. The authors of the review stated the following conclusions:

> "Although a number of studies suggest that TENS may produce short lived improvements in some neuropsychological or behavioural aspects of dementia, the limited presentation and availability of data from these studies does not allow definite conclusions on the possible benefits of this intervention. Since most of the currently published studies are well designed, although the numbers of subjects in each study is small, analysis of the complete original data from these and/or future studies may allow more definitive conclusions to be drawn."[34]

Behavior Management Techniques

Summary: The findings from three reviews provide some support for behavior management techniques as effective interventions for behavioral symptoms of dementia, though mixed study results, the variety of specific interventions, and methodological concerns in many studies suggest that, though behavior management techniques are promising interventions for the treatment of behavioral symptoms of dementia, additional research with carefully assessed outcomes is warranted to replicate results across research labs and settings.

Details: Behavior management techniques include a wide variety of behavioral interventions such as functional analysis of specific behaviors (e.g., establishing how behaviors or responses are influenced by stimuli), token economies (e.g., systems of positive reinforcement for behaviors), habit training (e.g., reinforced learning of habits related to activities of daily living), progressive muscle relaxation, communication training, behavioral or cognitive-behavioral therapy, and various types of individualized behavioral reinforcement strategies. These interventions can be implemented directly with the patient or taught to caregivers to implement with the patient.

Three good quality systematic reviews,[7, 11, 35] including a total of 31 studies, examined the effectiveness of behavior management techniques for the treatment of behavioral symptoms of dementia. An additional 11 articles focused on teaching caregivers to implement behavior management techniques with individuals with dementia. Of these 42 articles, seven were RCTs with sample sizes of more than 30 participants. The remaining studies were limited by methodological issues including small sample sizes (e.g., single subject design or very small samples of less than 10 participants per treatment condition), non-randomization, patients serving as their own comparison subjects, or no comparison group. Additionally, two primary studies not included in the three good quality reviews were examined for this report after recommendation by reviewers, resulting in a total of nine primary articles considered in this report. The two primary articles suggested by reviewers were both behavior management technique RCTs documenting some decreases in behavioral symptoms of dementia; the seven RCTs from the systematic reviews provided mixed evidence for the effectiveness of behavior management techniques. Table 1 shows the details of these nine studies.

Non-pharmacological Interventions for Behavioral Symptoms of Dementia

Table 1. Primary studies on behavior management techniques

Sample Size	Randomiz-ation	Blinding	Clustering/ Nesting	Type of Intervention and Comparator	Outcomes	Results
N=120 in matched care facilities Final N: treatment = 54, control = 51[36]	Yes: Random assignment to matched care facilities.	No blinding of providers or assessors; patients were "unaware whether their carer received the intervention or not."	Yes: Clustering accounted for by using generalized estimating equations.	Treatment: Staff training on "psychosocial management of residents' behavioral problems." Control: Treatment as usual.	Four behavioral outcome measures: AGECAT Organic, AGECAT Depression, Chrichton Scale, Barthel Index. Ten outcome measures of provider visits.	Pre-test group differences on AGECAT Organic once clustering was accounted for. Treatment group: Significant difference in AGECAT Organic and AGECAT Depression; significantly fewer general practitioner visits; no significant differences in nine other provider visit measures.
N = 72 dyads[2]	Yes: Random assignment to 1 of 4 conditions.	No provider blinding; yes assessor blinding; no patient blinding.	No clustering, just caregiver-patient dyads.	Treatment 1: Teaching caregivers to implement increased pleasant events; Treatment 2: Teaching caregivers problem solving strategies; Control 1: Typical care; Control 2: Waitlist.	HDRS, CSDD, BDI, MMSE, DRS, RIL, caregiver HDRS, BI, and ten items on positive aspects of care-giving.	Significant gender differences at pre-test but no differences on outcome measures; gender was included as a covariate but was not associated with outcomes. Immediate post-test: Significant improvement on all patient and caregiver depression measures for both treatment and neither control groups. No significant differences on any measures of cognition or burden, consistent with research hypotheses. Six month follow-up (only treatment groups assessed): Significant improvement in patient and caregiver depressions scores was maintained compared to pre-test.
N = 153 dyads[37]	Yes: Random assignment to treatment or control.	Yes assessor blinding; no provider blinding; no information on patient blinding.	No clustering, just caregiver-patient dyads.	Treatment: Patient exercise program combined with teaching caregivers behavior management which included general behavior management as well as education about dementia, moderating personal reactions, and identifying and encouraging pleasant activities including exercise and social activities. Control: Routine care.	SF-36-PF, SF-36-PRF, SIP-BCM, SIP-M, SIP-HM, HDRS, CSDD, walking speed, functional reach, standing balance, aerobic activity, restricted activity days, falls, near falls, RMBPC, MMSE.	No significant pre-test differences. Three months post test: Significant differences in SF-36-PRF, CDSS, aerobic activity, and restricted activity days. 24 months post-test: Significant differences in SF-36-PRF and SIP-M.
N = 95 dyads[38]	Yes: Random assignment to treatment or control.	Yes assessor blinding; no provider blinding; no information on patient blinding.	No clustering, just caregiver-patient dyads.	Treatment: Training consultants to teach caregivers behavior management techniques, communication, and pleasant events; and provide caregiver support. Control: Routine care.	Caregiver outcomes: CES-D, HDRS, CSQ, PSS, SCB, SSCQ. Patient outcomes: 3 caregiver-rated target behaviors, NPI, RMBPC, QOL-AD, MMSE.	Significant differences in ethnicity at baseline but unrelated to outcome. Post-test: Significant differences in CES-D, SCB, RMBPC, and QOL-AD. Six month follow-up: significant differences in CES-D, HDRS, CSQ, SCB, RMBPC, and QOL-AD.
N = 31 residents and 25 staff[39]	Yes: Random assignment to treatment or control.	Yes assessor blinding; no provider blinding; no information on patient blinding.	Yes: 4 residences in the RCT. Stats accounted for clustering by use of Huber-White-Sandwich estimator.	Training: Behavior management training of staff at residences. Control: Trainings as usual.	GDS, CAS, RMBPS, ABID, NPI, SSCQ, job satisfaction, MMSE.	No significant pre-test differences. Significant improvement in GDS, CAS, RMBPS, ABID, NPI.

Non-pharmacological Interventions for Behavioral Symptoms of Dementia

Sample Size	Randomization	Blinding	Clustering/ Nesting	Type of Intervention and Comparator	Outcomes	Results
N = 237 dyads[40]	Yes: Random assignment to treatment or control.	Yes: Providers, assessors, and patients blinded to condition.	No clustering, just caregiver-patient dyads.	Treatment: Training caregivers on problem solving, communication, engaging patients in activities, and simplifying tasks. Control: Phone calls using a script focusing on care challenges and informational brochures.	Patient outcomes: FIM-IADL, FIM-ADL, QOL-AD, Activity engagement scale, ABID. Caregiver outcomes: PCI, caregiver confidence scale, behavior problems, study benefits.	No significant pre-test differences. 4 month follow-up: Significant improvement in FIM-IADL, Activity engagement, PCI, and caregiver confidence. 9 month follow-up: No significant differences on any outcome measure.
N = 127[41]	Yes: Random assignment to 1 of 5 treatment or control groups.	No information provided but likely no provider blinding.	5 treatment and control groups at each of 7 sites; statistics accounted for differences by state but not site.	Treatment groups: (1) ADL, (2) Psychosocial activities, and (3) Combined ADL/Activities. Control groups: (1) Placebo of 30 minutes daily nursing assistant attention and (2) treatment as usual.	DBS, MMSE, ODAS, AARS, and VAS.	No significant pre-test differences. Significant differences on some subscales of the ODAS, AARS, and VAS though total number of subscales was not reported.
N = 34 dyads[42]	Yes: Random assignment to treatment or control.	No information provided but likely no provider blinding.	No clustering, just caregiver-patient dyads.	Treatment: Progressive muscle relaxation (PMR). Control: Imagery intervention matched to PMR for provider contact, time, structure, assessment, and home practice.	BVRT, COWA, CF, BAI, MBPC, BRAD, DRS, BPRS.	No significant pre-test differences. Post-test significant improvement in BVRT, COWA, CF, MBPC, BPRS, and BRAD.
N = 57 dyads in 5 care facilities[43]	Yes: Random assignment to treatment or control.	No patient or family member blinding; nursing staff blinded by being kept uninformed of study hypotheses.	Treatment was provided in groups held within 5 care facilities; no statistical accounting for clustering.	Treatment: Caregiver training on verbal communication, non-verbal communication, and family visit structure. Control: Usual care (no comparable group participation).	Patient outcomes: MOSES-Self-care, MOSES-Disorientation, MOSES-Depression, MOSES-Irritability, MOSES-Withdrawal, CSDD-Mood-related signs, CSDD-Behavioral disturbance, CSDD-Physical signs, CSDD-Cyclic functions, CSDD-Ideational disturbance, CMAI-O-Physically aggressive, CMAI-O-Verbally agitated, CMAI-O-Physically nonaggressive, CMAI-N-Physically aggressive, CMAI-N-Nonaggressive, CMAI-N-Verbally agitated, GIPB-Verbal Behavior, GIPB-Nonverbal behavior, GIPB-Non-interactive behavior, MBP, psychotropic medication, restraint use. Family member outcomes: DMSS-Criticism, DMSS-Encouragement, DMSS-Active management, CHS-M-ADL, CHS-M-IADL, CHS-M-Behavior Problems, CHS-M-Cognitive functioning, CHS-M-Social network, VSO-Frequency of visit, VSO-Duration of visit, VSO-Amount of communication, VSO-Quality of communication, VSO-Impact on family members, VSO-Impact on residents.	Pre-test differences based on gender and length of stay accounted for statistically. 3-month follow-up: Significant improvement on MOSES-Disorientation, CSDD-Physical signs, CSDD-Cyclic functions, CSDD-Ideational disturbance, GIPB-Verbal behavior, GIPB-Non-interactive behavior, psychotropic medication, restraint use, DMSS-Criticism, and DMSS-Encouragement. 6-month follow-up: Significant improvement on MOSES-Depression, MOSES-Irritability, CSDD-Cyclic functions, CSDD-Ideational disturbance, CMAI-O-Verbally agitated, CMAI-N-Nonaggressive, DMSS-Criticism, CHS-Cognitive functioning, VSO-Duration of visit, and VSO-Impact on residents.

Abbreviations are defined in Appendix F.

There are a number of methodological concerns that affect the confidence of any estimate of effect in these studies, and the ability to clearly discern a pattern of effect across studies. One concern was inadequate blinding to treatment condition: in almost all reviewed studies, one or more key personnel (patients, caregivers, assessors, staff member raters, or providers) were not blinded to treatment condition; Gitlin et al. (2010) was the only study to document adequate double blinding.[40] The issue of adequate blinding is particularly important in these types of behavior management technique studies because almost all outcomes are assessed by provider or caregiver observation or patient self-report measures, all potentially influenced by provider or patient awareness of treatment condition.

Another important recurrent issue was the striking variation in the types of outcomes assessed and methods of outcome assessment (Table 1). Though all primary studies cited improvements in outcomes from behavior management interventions, many used multiple tools to measure the same construct (e.g., three depression scales in one study) but did not find consistent results within the study. Moreover, studies investigated a large number and variety of patient outcomes, including behavioral symptoms, depression, anxiety, psychiatric symptoms, cognitive functioning, activities of daily living, instrumental activities of daily living, aspects of physical health, quality of life, and activity participation. The inclusion of too many outcomes, especially in studies with smaller sample size, increases the likelihood that chance alone will produce a beneficial effect on one or more outcomes (i.e., increased risk of a Type I error or false alarm rate). For example, McCallion et al. (1999) acknowledge that the inclusion of multiple outcome measures assessed at both three- and six-months post-treatment resulted in an increased Type I error rate.[43] Though they used a more conservative p value (significance value) in their discussion of findings, the reported 21 significant outcomes out of a total of 68 assessed outcomes at various time points yielded inconsistent results within assessed constructs (e.g., patients improved on only certain measures assessing aggression, and they improved at only one time point on certain measures assessing affect).

Intervention characteristics also varied among studies, which in part reflects the diversity of interventions that fall under the behavior management therapy category such as functional analysis of specific behaviors, token economies, habit training, progressive muscle relaxation, communication training, behavioral or cognitive-behavioral therapy, and various types of individualized behavioral reinforcement strategies. Additionally, because behavior management techniques are often rooted in patient-specific behavior change, standardized interventions often used particular reinforcement strategies that varied from patient to patient.

This variability in outcomes, assessment tools, and interventions results in a body of literature that is difficult to compare, and it is almost impossible to establish specific, effective components of interventions that are broadly classified as behavior management techniques. Additionally, findings across studies were inconsistent even when similar interventions and outcomes were being assessed. Specific study findings are as follows:

- Proctor et al. (1999) found that an intervention training staff members in the psychosocial management of behavioral symptoms had positive effects on cognitive functioning and depression, yet there were no differences in physical disability or behavioral symptoms between the treatment and control groups.[36]

- Teri, Logsdon, et al. (1997) found that interventions designed to teach caregivers to implement problem solving strategies and increase pleasant events resulted in decreased depression; there was no change on measures of cognition.[44]

- Teri, Gibbons, et al. (2003) found that teaching caregivers behavior management techniques combined with a patient exercise program was effective in improving some aspects of patient physical health and depression, though these findings were inconsistent across measurement occasions.[45]

- Teri, McCurry, et al. (2005) found that training consultants to teach caregivers how to implement behavior management techniques and increase pleasant events resulted in a decrease in four out of seven measures of behavioral symptoms, quality of life, and psychiatric symptoms at post-test, and seven out of seven measures at six-month follow-up.[38]

- Teri, Huda, et al. (2005) examined a behavior management training program for assisted living facility staff and found that this intervention decreased all assessed patient outcomes in the treatment group including depression, anxiety, and behavioral symptoms.[39]

- Gitlin et al. (2010) found that a patient-tailored intervention program targeting problem solving, communication, engagement in activities, and task restructuring resulted in significant improvements in functional independence and quality of life, as well as some improvements in agitated behaviors and engagement in activities; these latter findings were inconsistent across post-test and nine-month follow-up assessment periods.[40]

- Beck et al. (2002) investigated an intervention focused on activities of daily living and psychosocial activities; these interventions resulted in some improvements in patient affect, though no improvements in patient disruptive behaviors were noted.[41]

- Suhr et al. (1999) found that a progressive muscle relaxation intervention resulted in significant improvement in behavioral symptoms and cognitive functioning, and no change in anxiety.[42]

- McCallion et al. (1999) found that an intervention designed to improve caregiver-patient communication resulted in improvements on some measures of depression and behavioral symptoms, though these findings were inconsistent across measurement occasions.[43]

The three reviews on behavior management techniques examined a broader range of primary studies than the subset of primary articles included in this report due to the methodological concerns of the studies. In spite of including a broader range of primary studies, these reviews document cautious recommendations for the effectiveness of behavior management techniques in the treatment of behavioral symptoms of dementia. Ayalon et al. (2006)[7] described the interventions as possibly efficacious, and noted the need for replication and further research; Logsdon et al. (2007)[35] described two effective behavior management techniques, structured behavioral interventions and individualized interventions designed to target behavioral symptoms, as being effective in the treatment of dementia-related behavior symptoms; finally, Livingston et al. (2005)[11] used the Oxford Centre for Evidence-Based Medicine criteria[46] and rated behavior management techniques with a grade of B for the management of neuropsychiatric symptoms of dementia, noting that the larger RCTs for behavior management techniques that were reviewed resulted in consistently positive results even months following the interventions.

Neither the implementation of behavior management techniques with patients nor the teaching of behavior management techniques to caregivers to administer to patients was associated with any harm in any of the reviews or primary studies considered in this report, though this was not systematically assessed in the majority of studies.

Other Psychosocial Interventions

Animal-assisted Therapy (AAT)

Summary: Though some benefit of AAT on behavioral symptoms is suggested by the authors of these studies, this is a very limited body of evidence. Most studies were not experimental, did not have adequate control groups, had small sample sizes, and lacked methodological rigor. There were no RCTs. Moreover, no study performed a rigorous evaluation of feasibility, safety, cost, and staff training required to implement pet therapy in long-term care facilities.

Details: In 2006, the British National Institute for Health and Clinical Excellence (NICE) published guidelines for supporting people with dementia and their caretakers in health and social care.[4] The guidelines promoted the use of pet therapy as a non-verbal treatment for patients with verbal impairment, and also advocated pet therapy for patients requiring individualized treatment plans based on preferences, skills, and abilities.[4]

Our initial search for systematic reviews identified no previously published reviews of AAT for dementia. We conducted a search for primary studies and identified nine relevant studies that used quasi-experimental or repeated-measure within-participant designs (Table 2). The largest study included 62 subjects, and four of the studies enrolled 15 or fewer subjects. There were no RCTs.

These studies examined a broad range of AATs. One small study (n=9) examined the effects of two 10-minute interactive sessions, one with a robotic cat and one with a plush toy cat, and found that agitation decreased significantly among its participants when they held a plush toy cat.[47] Another small study (n=6) compared 10-minute sessions with a live cat versus a toy cat, and found that live cats increased meaningful communication, which suggests that patients with dementia may benefit from external stimuli to encourage dialogue.[48] A third study (n=20) compared the effects of pet therapy with traditional recreation therapy in treating passivity and reported that AAT participants were significantly more engaged and motivated to interact with their environment. Mood and patient satisfaction also significantly improved in the AAT group.[49] The presence of a resident dog among 22 nursing home residents was associated with decreased scores on all subscales of the Nursing Home Behavior Problem Scale during the day shift of the study but not during the evening hours.[50] The presence of a fish aquarium was associated with increased nutritional intake among individuals with Alzheimer's disease as well as reduced wandering in some individuals.[51]

Table 2. Studies of animal-assisted therapy

Setting	Subjects (n)	Behavioral Symptoms Addressed	Measures	Intervention	Findings
Rural nursing homes[49]	n=20; 15 females, 5 males; mean age was 78.9 years	Attention, mood, engagement, passivity	Dementia Mood Picture; Passivity in Dementia Scale; Resident Satisfaction Survey	10 participants received AAT; 10 participants received traditional recreation therapy. Data collection: pre (about mood), during (observational data), and post (participant satisfaction). Author did not list how many sessions were included nor how long the study lasted.	Mood and satisfaction significantly and positively changed for the AAT treatment group (p=0.03). AAT treatment group participants were found to be more engaged (p=0.002) and motivated to interact with environment (p=0.006). Reduction of passivity was the overall finding.
Large, suburban not-for-profit nursing home[47]	n=9; All were female, mean age was 90 years	Agitation, pleasure, interest, sadness, anxiety, anger, attention, attitude, intensity of manipulation with the stimuli, engagement	Agitated Behaviors Mapping Instrument (ABMI); Lawton's Modified Behavior Stream; 5-point scale (attention, attitude, manipulation); Minutes (duration of engagement)	2 interactive sessions, lasting 10 minutes each on different days – 1 with robotic cat and 1 with plush toy cat. Presentation of cats to participants was randomized.	The plush toy cat resulted in a significant decrease of overall agitation (p=0.036) and physically disrupted behavior. The robotic cat yielded a significant increase in pleasure (p=0.007). The intensity of manipulation with the robotic cat was higher than with the plush cat (p=0.081). Only 22 percent of participants held the robotic cat, whereas 78 percent held the plush cat.
Special care unit of two nursing homes[52]	n=15; 14 female, 1 male; mean age was 86.8 years	Agitation classified in three syndromes: physically aggressive behaviors, physically nonaggressive behaviors, verbally agitated behaviors. Social behaviors assessed.	Cohen-Mansfield Agitation Inventory (CMAI); Mini-Mental State Examination (MMSE); AAT (animal-assisted therapy) flow sheet; Record of PRN medication	Daily AAT sessions with visiting dog for 3 weeks. Data collected at baseline, at the end of the 3-week intervention, and 3 weeks after the intervention ended.	Therapeutic recreation AAT intervention shown to decrease agitated behaviors (p=0.001) and increase social interactions (p=0.009).
Three dementia-specific units located in extended-care facilities[51]	n=62; 24 males, 38 females, mean age was 80.1 years	Nutritional intake	Nutritional intake was recorded as the difference in grams	For 6 weeks, treatment facilities viewed aquariums. For 2 weeks, control facility viewed a scenic ocean picture, then pictures were removed for 2 weeks (washout period), then facility received aquarium for 2 weeks.	Nutritional intake increased significantly in the presence of aquariums (p<0.001). Some participants with a history of pacing and wandering were found to sit for longer periods. Participants were observed to be more attentive and awake. Nutritional supplements decreased due to the increase in nutritional intake.
Special care unit of an urban extended healthcare facility[50]	n=22; 15 females, 7 males; mean age was 83.7 years	Aggressive, irrational, sleep, inappropriate, annoying, & dangerous behaviors	Medication review form; Nursing Home Behavior Problem Scale (NHBPS)	Behavioral symptoms were documented 1 week before introduction of dog and weekly for 4 weeks following placement of dog.	Presence of the resident dog decreased behavioral symptoms during the daytime hours (p<0.05), but there were no significant differences during the evening hours.

Non-pharmacological Interventions for Behavioral Symptoms of Dementia

Setting	Subjects (n)	Behavioral Symptoms Addressed	Measures	Intervention	Findings
Nursing home[48]	n=6; all female; ranged in age from 84 to 90	Verbal communication	Mini Mental Status Examination (MMSE); Functional Assessment Tool for Alzheimer's-Type Dementia (FAST); verbal communication measures	3 10-minute baseline, withdrawal and intervention phases with half of the participants receiving the live cat first and half receiving the toy cat first.	Study revealed that the live cats have the greatest influence on all measures, which included number of total words, meaningful information units (MIU), and initiations. Overall, there was an increase in meaningful communication with the live cats present based on total word count.
Three special care units of extended care facilities[53]	n=28; 21 females, 7 males; mean age was 83.8	Agitation, socialization	Burke Dementia Behavioral Rating Scale (BDBRS); Agitation Behavior Mapping Instrument (ABMI); Daubenmire's Data Coding Protocol (DDCP)	6 observation sessions that included videotaping participants for 15 seconds every 5 minutes. 2 30-minute sessions were conducted with or without the dog present.	Positive changes in agitation and socialization were observed (e.g., increase in verbalizations, smiles, looks, leans, and tactile contact). Decreased agitation was also found. P-values were not provided.
Three long-term care facilities[54]	n=22; 12 females, 10 males; mean age was 77.9 years	Social interaction variables and physiological variables	Burke Dementia Scale; Heart rate; Blood pressure; Mean arterial pressure; Peripheral skin temperature	10-minute sessions were held on 2 different days; 1 day with and 1 day without the dog present – held in a private room. Randomization was used to assign the order of the sessions.	The presence of the therapy dog enhanced nonverbal communication and increased socialization behaviors: frequency of smiles ($p<0.05$) and duration of smiles ($p<0.01$); frequency of looks ($p<0.05$); duration of looks ($p<0.01$); frequency of tactile contact ($p<0.01$) and duration of tactile contact ($p<0.01$).
Special care Alzheimer's unit of a large Midwest Veterans home[55]	n=12; 2 females, 10 males; ranged in age from 66 to 88 years old	Social behaviors (8 categories)	Social behaviors observation checklist	5-minute observation sessions at baseline (pretreatment without dog); when dog was temporarily present (weekly dog visits); and 2 weeks after the dog became a permanent resident for a total of 6 observation sessions.	Significant increase in more social behaviors ($p<0.001$) with dog present; found no difference between visiting and resident dog or between individual and group settings.

Exercise

Summary: This body of literature shows inconsistent results of exercise interventions on behavioral symptoms and functional status. Variations in intensity of exercise intervention, severity of dementia at baseline and outcome measures make it difficult to draw a firm conclusion. Many of the included studies were small and did not use rigorous methodology. The most consistent evidence showed that exercise did increase sleep duration and decrease nighttime awakenings. While the impact of improved sleep on distal health outcomes remains uncertain, there may be an additional benefit to caregivers who are disproportionally affected by dysfunctional sleep.

Details: We identified three systematic reviews on the effects of physical activity programs for dementia.[56-58]

A Cochrane review aimed to determine whether physical activity programs maintained or improved cognition, function, behavior, depression and/or mortality when compared to usual care in persons with dementia.[56] The review included randomized controlled trials of older adults with a dementia diagnosis who were allocated to either physical activity or usual care groups. Trials in which the exercise intervention was paired with another intervention were excluded.

The search identified four studies that met methodological quality criteria. The patients in the four included studies all carried a diagnosis of dementia and resided in the community or in long-term care facilities. The interventions varied broadly in intensity, frequency and duration. Three of these trials evaluated the effects of exercise on behavior, using validated scales to measure activities such as wandering, active aggression, and restlessness.[59-61] The fourth trial evaluated function but not behavior.[62] The authors were only able to combine data from two studies in a meta-analysis and found no effect of exercise on behavioral outcomes.

The Cochrane review was the most restrictive in its inclusion criteria among the reviews on exercise, and found insufficient evidence for drawing conclusions about the efficacy of exercise on behavioral and functional outcomes. The reviewers noted methodological shortcomings in the published literature and also noted other possible explanations for the lack of significant findings, including small sample size, quality of the intervention, poor adherence to the interventions, and differences in population characteristics.[56]

Another systematic review by Eggermont et al. (2006) took a broader approach by including non-randomized controlled trials; studies in which participants had varying degrees of cognitive impairment; studies in which exercise was the primary intervention (but could be combined with another intervention); and studies in which outcomes assessed included behavior, mood, sleep, or functional ability.[57] After a comprehensive search of studies published between 1974 and 2005, the review found 27 studies that met their inclusion and exclusion criteria, for a total participant sample size of 1,160. Out of 27 studies evaluated, their review included only six RCTs that had clearly defined outcome measures, clearly defined inclusion and exclusion criteria, adequate allocation concealment, and accounting for drop outs. The other included studies were lacking at least one of these criteria. The authors then grouped all included studies by outcome measures and evaluated the effects of exercise on behavior in terms of affect, sleep, and activities of daily living.

Seventeen of the 27 studies discuss the effect of exercise on affective behavior. Five were randomized controlled trials (RCTs), and the other 12 were poorer quality RCTs or observational studies. Two of the RCTs found exercise improved affective behaviors such as depression and agitation.[63, 64] The other three RCTs evaluating affective behavior showed neutral results.[65-67] Eggermont et al. (2006) explained this inconsistency by noting that the two positive studies used walking as part of the intervention, while the others used mostly seated strengthening exercises.

Six of the 27 studies examined the effect of exercise on sleep. Three of these were good quality RCTs which evaluated an intensive exercise intervention and used wrist sleep monitors to measure sleep.[63, 64, 67] All had positive results with increased nighttime sleep, decreased daytime sleep, and decreased awakenings. In fact, all studies showed a positive effect on sleep except for one prospective cohort trial which had neutral results. In this study, participants had minimal sleep disturbances at baseline, which may explain the lack of improvement.

Six of the 27 studies evaluated the effects of physical activity on functional ability. There was one good quality randomized control trial that showed improvements in ADLs, balance, timed get up and go, and a physical performance test.[68] Among the additional five studies that looked at functional ability, only one showed a positive result and this was only in the participants who were most dysfunctional at baseline. The authors note that each of these five trials used interventions of shorter duration compared with the positive RCT.

Overall, Eggermont et al.'s (2006) review[57] includes a wider range of trials that were of varying quality compared to the Cochrane review.[56] Though a number of studies found that exercise improved affective and functional outcomes, the overall strength of this conclusion is limited by inconsistencies among trials. On the other hand, a moderate body of consistent evidence showed that exercise programs can improve sleep in persons with dementia. Using the higher quality studies to make their conclusions, the reviewers posited that exercise activities that included walking were more likely to have a positive effect on mood compared to interventions without, and that frequent exercise sessions were more likely to lead to improvements in sleep compared to more sporadic sessions. Interventions of longer duration may have a benefit on functional ability in dementia patients. The authors also note that impairments in affective, functional, and sleep outcomes can have a disproportionate impact on caregivers, yet most of these studies did not evaluate outcomes such as caregiver satisfaction, which may be an important direction for future research in this field.

In a third systematic review on exercise and dementia, Heyn et al. (2004) opted to take a more quantitative approach and conducted a meta-analysis of the effects of physical exercise on dementia.[58] The analysis included RCTs of older patients with dementia as defined by MMSE scores or a physician diagnosis. Studies were excluded if they did not contain enough statistical information to compute an effect size, or if outcomes other than those specified were evaluated. Thirty trials were found that met these criteria, and they were grouped by outcome including cardiovascular fitness, strength, flexibility, Body Mass Index (BMI), functional status, cognition, and behavior.

The meta-analysis found significant heterogeneity in the data which may have led to inaccurate conclusions. While Heyn et al. (2004) used rigorous methodology in their search, little descriptive information was provided regarding the types of exercise interventions and the outcome measures. Moreover, it is difficult to translate the effect size determined by this review into real life outcomes. The overall results suggest that exercise has a positive effect on dementia patients' functional and behavioral status, but the details remain elusive.

Various Interventions Targeting a Specific Behavioral Symptom

Wandering

Summary: Overall, quality evidence is lacking to determine if subjective barriers prevent or reduce wandering by cognitively impaired people in an institutional or domestic setting, and possible adverse effects remain unknown. There is insufficient evidence to draw any conclusions about the effectiveness of multisensory stimulation, exercise, therapeutic touch, aromatherapy, or music therapy for wandering among patients with dementia. Uncontrolled studies suggest that GPS location systems for wandering behavior may improve patient safety. More rigorous trials are needed to assess the feasibility and effectiveness of these devices in broader use within VA.

Details: The wandering behavior of cognitively impaired people presents risk and places additional demands on caretakers. The prevalence of wandering by people with dementia is difficult to assess. Wandering is not a simple or static behavior, and the reasons why people wander remain unclear: The same behavior or types of wandering might occur for different reasons in different individuals.[69] Traditional measures to reduce wandering include drugs, restraints, locked doors, and other barriers; but such interventions can be harmful.[70] It has been hypothesized that non-pharmacological treatments for wandering may provide safe and ethical alternatives.

We located five systematic reviews that focused on interventions for wandering.[69-73] Two publications by the same authors represent the same body of work: one is a journal article [72] based on a comprehensive report compiled for the Health Technology Assessment Program of the UK National Health Service.[71] The reviews included studies of a variety of interventions including subjective barriers, wandering in the domestic setting, and multiple interventions for the treatment of wandering.

One review conducted by the Cochrane Collaboration examined the use of subjective barriers, defined as barriers that appear as an obstruction only to persons with cognitive impairment. Examples of subjective barriers include mirrors, floor stripes or grids, camouflage of doors or doorknobs, and concealment of view through door windows. The literature review sought to identify RCTs on the use of subjective barriers but found no available RCTs. The authors therefore concluded that evidence evaluating the effect of subjective barriers is lacking, and the possibility that such barriers cause psychological harm remains unknown.[70]

Another Cochrane review sought to examine interventions for wandering of people with dementia in the domestic setting, as opposed to the institutional setting.[69] Although the literature search for RCTs found no RCTs conducted in the domestic setting, two RCTs conducted in institutional settings determined that exercise and walking therapies had no impact on wandering. The review also described the growing interest in the use of wander gardens in long-term care settings, but that the effects of such gardens on wandering behaviors are largely anecdotal.[69]

A third systematic review[71] on wandering examined the effectiveness of a variety of non-pharmacological interventions for wandering and included 11 studies (N=594), of which 8 were RCTs. Interventions for wandering included multisensory stimulation, exercise, therapeutic touch, aromatherapy, and music. Range of follow-up was three days to one year, with a mean duration of six weeks. The pooled results of two multisensory stimulation (MSS) studies showed a small, significant reduction in scores for restlessness 10 minutes after the intervention. Results of an exercise intervention showed a significant reduction in wandering in one study, but standard deviation scores were not reported and, therefore, results should be interpreted with caution. One of three studies focusing on therapeutic touch found a significant decrease in pacing but not on wandering or escaping from restraints. One study found that patients who received essential oils (type of oil not listed) compared to a control oil showed a decrease in wandering (P=0.05), while an additional study reported no significant difference in wandering behavior compared to controls. Music therapy showed no effect on wandering behavior. Overall, it is inconclusive as to whether multisensory stimulation, exercise, therapeutic touch, aromatherapy, or music therapy has a measurable effect on the behavioral symptoms of wandering associated with dementia.

A descriptive review of information and communication technology (ICT) devices identified 13 interventions that focused largely on wandering behaviors.[73] These examples of smart home technologies included Global Positioning System (GPS) location systems, boundary alarms activated by wristband, floor-lighting systems activated upon wandering detection, communication systems instructing the patient to return to bed after failure to return for a pre-defined period of time, and alarms alerting the caregiver of wandering behavior. The evidence consisted of case studies; cross-sectional studies; or single-group, pre- and post-test/post-test only studies. The settings included residential homes, nursing homes, and hospital settings. The devices were generally found to be effective, reliable, and successful in detecting wandering, locating lost patients, and reducing patient and caregiver stress. The intervention studies were generally limited in design by the lack of a control group, or by lack of blinding when a control group was used. Uncontrolled studies suggest that GPS location systems for wandering behavior may improve patient safety. More rigorous trials are needed to assess the feasibility and effectiveness of these devices in broader use within VA.

Agitation

Summary: Overall, there is no evidence demonstrating an effect of social contact, environmental modification, caregiver training, combination therapy, or behavior therapy on the behavioral symptoms of agitation in dementia. A weak body of evidence suggests sensory interventions may improve agitation. One recent primary study provides preliminary evidence suggesting that systematic individualized intervention may be effective in improving the symptom of agitation, though additional evidence is needed.

Details: Agitation is defined as an inappropriate verbal, vocal, or motor activity that is not explained by needs or confusion.[74] We found one review that focused on the behavioral symptoms of agitation for dementia.[74] The review identified 14 randomized trials (combined number of subjects=586) that included six types of intervention: sensory interventions, social contact, environmental modification, caregiver training, combination therapy, and behavior therapy. Study designs included randomized controlled parallel and randomized cross-over study designs, and usual care constituted the comparator in each study. The duration of treatment ranged across studies from ten minutes to one year. Four studies included follow-up at longer than two months and were thus able to examine the long-term effects of interventions. In addition to the one review, we included one recently conducted primary study suggested to us by reviewers.

Among the seven types of interventions tested in the studies included in the review, sensory interventions (aromatherapy, thermal bath, calming music, and hand massage) were found to be effective: pooled data from three studies (N=120), which included two RCTs and one randomized cross-over design (RCO), showed a statistically significant decrease in agitation between treatment groups and control groups. These findings should be interpreted with caution, however. Several factors limit the conclusions that can be drawn from the pooled findings: there was a small number of studies in each intervention category; there was substantial variability in the duration of the intervention programs (including one study that used a single 10-minute exposure) and outcome measures used; and the definitions of agitation were inconsistent across studies.

Of the four studies that tested long-term effects (> 2-month follow-up) of interventions, there were no significant differences in agitation between treatment groups and control groups for caregiver training, combination therapy, and behavioral therapy.[74]

One primary study was included based on reviewer feedback. This study documented a randomized, placebo-controlled trial of a systematic individualized intervention designed to target the symptom of agitation.[75] The authors described a decision tree intervention model designed to target unmet needs in individuals exhibiting agitation; therefore, the intervention was individualized to participants and included a potentially unlimited variety of specific intervention strategies. The systematic individualized intervention was described as a decision tree model to assist providers and caregivers in identifying unmet needs that could cause behavioral symptoms of dementia, and the individually tailored treatments were left to the discretion of the care professional. Examples of specific treatments that were implemented included altering the environment for increased familiarity and comfort, engagement in meaningful activities, and using safety devices. Participants were 167 residents in 12 nursing homes. Randomization was at the level of nursing home, with six nursing homes receiving the treatment condition and six receiving the placebo control. The study was randomized and included a strong placebo control condition (i.e., the control condition consisted of an educational intervention to assure that control group staff was unaware of control group status). The authors do not adequately describe blinding procedures, however, and it appears as though raters who assessed agitation were not blind to treatment condition. Therefore, though this research provides preliminary results supporting the use of systematic individualized intervention to treat the symptom of agitation, these findings must be interpreted with caution due to the possibility of inadequate blinding which could affect the validity of the study.

Inappropriate Sexual Behavior

There were no systematic reviews that examined the topic of inappropriate sexual behavior among individuals with dementia. Currently, the effectiveness of non-pharmacological treatments for inappropriate sexual behavior remains unknown.

Comparative Effectiveness among Non-pharmacological Interventions and between Pharmacological and Non-pharmacological Approaches

None of the systematic reviews captured in our search identified any head-to-head trials that directly compared effectiveness among different non-pharmacological interventions, or between non-pharmacological and pharmacological treatments.

One systematic review compared the effect sizes from studies of non-pharmacological interventions to separate studies of cholinesterase inhibitors.[76] The review identified studies of the effects of bright light therapy, physical activity, tactile stimulation, and the use of cholinesterase inhibitors (donepezil, galantamine, rivastigmine, and tacrine) on cognition, affective behavior, and sleep-wake rhythm in persons with dementia. The review attempted to quantify pooled effect sizes for each form of intervention, although the analysis was limited by substantial heterogeneity between studies and inadequate reporting of methodology. The review determined that the effect sizes were similar between non-pharmacological interventions and cholinesterase inhibitors on cognition and affective behavior.[76]

KEY QUESTION #2. How do non-pharmacological treatments of behavioral symptoms compare in safety with each other, with pharmacological approaches, and with no treatment?

Cognitive/Emotion-oriented Interventions

None of the systematic reviews included in this report identified direct evidence on the adverse effects of reminiscence therapy or validation therapy. One study found that simulated presence therapy increased agitation and disruptive behaviors in some patients, while decreasing agitation in others.[3] In one study of validation therapy, reality orientation was used as a comparator intervention.[14] The Health Technology Assessment (HTA) report[71] noted three studies in which professional and non-professional caregivers found that reality orientation could actually increase distress, fear, and agitation in the person with dementia and, therefore, was not deemed to be an acceptable strategy to manage behavior. In a qualitative study component of the HTA review, caregivers conveyed that reality orientation may be more useful in the earlier stages of dementia, but for people in the later stages, reality orientation could cause great distress for some individuals. Staff caregivers preferred to tell "white lies" than answer some direct questions and risk upsetting residents.

Sensory Stimulation Interventions

The systematic reviews that we included on the use of acupuncture, aromatherapy, light therapy, massage/touch, music therapy, Snoezelen multisensory stimulation, and TENS did not identify direct evidence on safety of these interventions in individuals with dementia. The HTA report noted that with sensory stimulation therapies such as music therapy and massage/touch therapy, not all individuals respond favorably to the treatment, and the increased stimulus could increase agitation and aggression in some individuals.[71]

Behavior Management Techniques

The three systematic reviews included in this report did not specifically address the safety or potential harm of any behavior management techniques. None of the nine RCTs reviewed for this report included direct evidence on potential harm, though none documented any patient harm or adverse events that occurred with the implementation of the techniques. Because of the variety of interventions included in this area as well as the individualized implementation strategies often utilized in the administration of behavior management techniques, it is theoretically possible that certain types of interventions have the potential to cause harm (e.g., the use of risky or dangerous reinforcement strategies).

Other Psychosocial Interventions

Animal-assisted Therapy

Although we found no studies addressing the safety of animal-assisted therapy, the guidelines of the American Veterinary Medical Association describe potential physical and emotional harms associated with animal-assisted therapy.[77] Human injury can result because of lack of supervision, inadequate participant training, or inappropriate handling. Zoonotic disease transmission is also of concern any time animals and humans interact, and can pose a threat to high-risk populations if good hygiene is not utilized. Moreover, participants can have potential allergic reactions to animal dander or saliva. Emotional risks for patients include grief or guilt should a therapy animal pass away. Program participants may become possessive of the animals, creating an atmosphere of competition rather than social well-being. Patients may perceive that an animal has rejected them, and the interaction could potentially exacerbate mood or behavioral symptoms.[77]

Exercise

Few studies discussed adverse events. Potential harms of exercise programs include the increased risk of falls or other adverse outcomes.

Various Interventions Targeting a Specific Behavioral Symptom

The HTA report noted the potential risk of a false sense of security in the caregiver associated with the use of tagging/tracking devices for wandering. Other systematic reviews included in our search did not identify evidence on adverse effects of interventions that target wandering or agitation.

Comparative Safety among Non-pharmacological Interventions and between Pharmacological and Non-pharmacological Approaches

None of the systematic reviews captured in our search identified any head-to-head trials that directly compared safety among different non-pharmacological interventions, or between non-pharmacological and pharmacological treatments.

KEY QUESTION #3. How do non-pharmacological treatments of behavioral symptoms compare in cost with each other, with pharmacological approaches, and with no treatment?

None of the systematic reviews we retrieved investigated or identified evidence on the cost-effectiveness of specific interventions. The HTA report on non-pharmacological interventions for wandering conducted a thorough literature search of economic studies or clinical studies containing relevant economic information, but found no studies that evaluated the cost-effectiveness of the interventions.[71] The HTA search identified literature on the tangible and intangible costs of behavioral symptoms in people with dementia, such as the additional resources posed by wandering behaviors or the additional hours spent caring, but the information was not specific to particular interventions.

Cost considerations for particular interventions are discussed below:

Animal-assisted Therapy

We found no studies on the costs of animal-assisted therapy, but the resources required for preparation, training, and care of a single animal for use in animal-assisted therapy are considerable. The therapeutic animal requires ongoing veterinary care, regular grooming, and individualized exercise; and liability and pet insurance are additional considerations. Some forms of animal-assisted therapy may have lower associated costs, such as the use of a visiting animal or the placement of aquariums in dining halls.

Tagging/Tracking Devices for Wandering

The HTA report noted the additional costs and resources associated with the use of tagging/tracking devices as a drawback to the feasibility of these interventions. The use of this technology requires extensive training and technical support, and places increased demand on informal caregivers in terms of using the equipment, monitoring, and searching for the care recipient.[71]

DISCUSSION

Overall, clear and consistent evidence supporting the use of the various psychosocial therapies for the treatment of behavioral symptoms for dementia is lacking. Many reviews reported mixed results with little consistent evidence either favoring or rejecting the intervention in question. There are few good quality RCTs and much of the evidence comes from small scale studies often with great variability in how behavioral symptoms are defined, duration of intervention, measuring instruments, and the outcome measures used to determine the effectiveness of the various interventions.

The literature seems to suggest that stimulation or sensory-oriented approaches (i.e., light therapy, aromatherapy, and massage/touch therapy) show greater promise than emotion-oriented approaches, but there is little data directly comparing these approaches and this finding should be interpreted with caution given the overall limitations in the bodies of evidence. The sensory-oriented approaches may be cost-effective and somewhat easy to implement within VA settings, particularly because many can be implemented by a variety of care-giving personnel without advanced degrees. For instance, aromatherapy and hand massage therapy may be implemented in a communal setting with little caregiver training and most likely without incurring a high treatment cost.[12]

None of the emotion-oriented approaches was well-studied. Program implementation for all three – validation therapy, reminiscence therapy, and simulated presence therapy – require master's level personnel.

There is some evidence to suggest that behavior management techniques are effective strategies to reduce behavioral symptoms of dementia (see Table 1); however, the results of the reviewed studies must be interpreted with caution due to methodological limitations. In particular, inadequate blinding, usual care rather than alternative treatment control groups, and multiple measured outcomes in the reviewed studies result in questionable findings in need of replication. Though multiple outcomes can be beneficial in detecting treatment effects, the comparable outcomes assessed across studies resulted in conflicting findings, suggesting that some positive outcomes might be due to chance. This body of research documents a wide variety of techniques that are often individualized to patients; though this is a methodological limitation in that it is difficult to compare interventions and determine effective components, it is also a potential strength of behavior management techniques. These techniques are flexible and adaptable to various settings and patients, lending themselves toward individual tailoring rather than to a standardized population approach. Additional research using standardized behavior management interventions is needed to replicate initial findings across research labs and with a variety of populations. Finally, preliminary research on behavior management technique training for care providers suggests that these techniques could be implemented in a variety of settings with providers who do not have advanced degrees; it is likely that, given additional research documenting the efficacy of specific training programs, such programs could be implemented in VA settings in a relatively cost-effective manner.

Exercise therapy was evaluated in a number of trials, though, again, variations in intervention dose and population studied make it difficult to offer generalizable conclusions about its effectiveness. Exercise did seem consistently to increase sleep time in individuals with dementia. Though findings were mixed for other outcomes, it is possible that an increase in sleep time may be an important benefit in and of itself for both patients and caregivers. Some data suggest regular exercise may help improve mobility and decrease the risk of falls, which might suggest a useful "by-product" of exercise programs for cognitively impaired adults.[78, 79] That cognitively impaired elderly adults are at increased risk of falls represents simultaneously a potential rationale for and risk of exercise programs. The proper intensity and frequency of exercise, along with the appropriate level of supervision required to minimize risk of falls, should be determined before exercise programs are implemented broadly in VA settings.

While it is important to evaluate the effectiveness of the various psychosocial interventions for behavioral symptoms of dementia with a wide range of participants and settings, it should be noted that there is also a need for individually tailored approaches. It is important to modify interventions to the specific needs and circumstances of the individuals with dementia, their caregivers, and their environment.[4] Given the lack of certainty of overall benefit from these interventions, implemented programs should strive to minimize associated harms. For example, though sensory-oriented approaches did appear to offer some benefit to some intervention participants, an increase in agitation may occur in other participants. Because individual participants may respond differently to treatment, an iterative, flexible approach to program development seems critical.[75] Some of the more recent studies investigating behavior management techniques[39] and systematic individualized interventions[75] provide preliminary evidence that targeted, tailored, and individualized approaches may be effective in decreasing certain behavioral symptoms of dementia; however, additional research replicated across research labs with adequate blinding of providers, raters, and participants is needed to strengthen this body of evidence.

There is much that remains unknown about the effectiveness and feasibility of non-pharmacological interventions. For instance, little is known about the potential harms from the various non-pharmacological treatments. Although the potential risk seems low, especially compared to the use of atypical and typical antipsychotic medication, few studies have included information on adverse events. Due to the potentially lesser risk associated with these techniques when compared with medication therapies, research documenting relative risk is warranted. In addition, as mentioned above, not all forms of psychosocial treatments for dementia may be appropriate for all patients. For example, simulated presence therapy has been shown to increase agitation and disruptive behaviors in some people while decreasing agitation in others.

Furthermore, it is unclear as to the extent to which patients may find certain therapies pleasurable in terms of duration and frequency. For instance, aromatherapy may be a pleasurable event when experienced for a short duration during a specific activity, but may cease to have an impact when patients are exposed on a continual basis or too frequently.

In addition, in cases where no treatment was used as the control, it is not clear if the simple act of receiving attention may have acted as a confounding variable. In other words, any additional form of attention may have an impact on the behavioral outcome in question and, thus, it is unknown if the intervention being tested produced the effect.

It is also unclear if these interventions can be used as a form of treatment for behavioral symptoms as opposed to prevention. Many of the interventions were performed during a predetermined time with an observer rating behavior before, during, and after the intervention. Thus, patients may not have been experiencing the behavior in question prior to the intervention. It is possible that the prevention of behavioral symptoms may be easier to address rather than intervening once patients start to experience behavioral symptoms. Further research is needed to determine the impact of non-pharmacological interventions on preventing and treating behavioral symptoms among persons with dementia.

FUTURE RESEARCH RECOMMENDATIONS

Overall, non-pharmacological treatments for the behavioral symptoms associated with dementia warrant further investigation in the form of large-scale RCTs of adequate duration. Several small studies suggest that some of the interventions (e.g., aromatherapy, music therapy, massage therapy, behavior management techniques, and animal-assisted therapy) may have potential benefits for individuals with dementia. Patients with dementia often have multiple behavioral symptoms associated with their disease (e.g., sleep awakening, aggression, wandering, and depression) that may respond to different interventions. Multi-component studies may be one way to address the multiple needs of patients with dementia.[80] Thus, a multi-component strategy to reduce the impact of behavioral symptoms should be included in further research.

Future studies should include RCTs with clearly defined interventions, with a focus on duration and frequency of the intervention as well as adverse effects. Validated tools should be used to measure outcomes; and adequate blinding of participants, raters, and providers is necessary to assure valid, replicable results. The cost-effectiveness, safety, and feasibility of interventions for implementation in VA settings need to be determined.

CONCLUSIONS

In conclusion, support for psychosocial interventions which effectively treat behavioral symptoms of dementia is mixed at best. For instance, one systematic review found that validation therapy fared better than usual care but produced no significant differences when compared to social contact or reality orientation for general behavioral symptoms. Validation therapy showed increased benefit compared to social contact for depression at 12-month follow-up, but it did no better than usual care or reality orientation. Findings from three additional reviews found no evidence that validation therapy reduces behavioral symptoms of dementia. The results were inconclusive for simulated presence therapy. One systematic review found that reminiscence therapy was better than no treatment for depression but was not significant in reducing behavioral symptoms, and additional reviews found no evidence to support the use of reminiscence therapy. The effectiveness of light therapy was also mixed, with one review suggesting there may be some benefit for agitation, nocturnal restlessness, and sleep disturbance. Aromatherapy shows some promise for reducing agitation but showed no improvement in aggression. Massage therapy fared better than no treatment in reducing agitation and disturbed behavior when compared to baseline but had no significant effect when compared to calming music. There is no available evidence to suggest that acupuncture is an effective treatment for behavioral symptoms, nor is there evidence that TENS reduces sleep disturbance or behavioral symptoms among patients with dementia. It remains unclear if subjective barriers, multisensory stimulation, exercise, therapeutic touch, aromatherapy, or music have an impact on wandering behavior. Agitation may be reduced by sensory interventions (i.e., aromatherapy, thermal bath, calming music, and hand massage); but there is currently no evidence to suggest that social contact, environmental modification, caregiver training, combination therapy, or behavior therapy is effective. There is preliminary evidence to suggest that systematic individualized intervention may be effective in reducing agitation, though this research is limited by methodology and therefore needs to be replicated with adequate blinding procedures to assure valid results. Finally, initial research on behavior management techniques is promising though inconsistent; methodologically rigorous replication studies utilizing adequate blinding procedures and standardized treatments across research labs and patient settings are needed to confirm the preliminary, positive results.

The summary of findings and quality of the evidence for each form of therapy is presented in Table 3. We defined the level of evidence using the definitions of the GRADE working group,[81] as follows:

- High – Further research is very unlikely to change our confidence in the estimate of effect;
- Moderate – Further research is likely to have an important impact on our confidence in the estimate of effect and may change the estimate;
- Low – Further research is very likely to have an important impact on our confidence in the estimate of effect and is likely to change the estimate;
- Very low – Any estimate of effect is very uncertain.

Non-pharmacological Interventions for Behavioral Symptoms of Dementia

Table 3. Summary of findings

Intervention	Studies included in Systematic Reviews (SRs)	Quality of data: Most recent search date Length of follow-up Consistency of findings	Estimate of benefit; overall level of evidence	Study limitations	Comments on feasibility and acceptability
Emotional Oriented Approaches					
Reminiscence Therapy	7 RCTs	Most recent search date: March 2006 Follow-up: ≥ 4 weeks Consistency of findings: Showed no benefit, except for depression in 1 small RCT	Neutral effect; low	Evidence is based on a small number of studies with very small sample sizes.	Requires a master's level counselor for implementation. Patients and caregivers appear to enjoy the intervention.
Simulated Presence Therapy (SPT)	1 RCT and 3 other studies	Most recent search date: February 2008 Follow-up: Not reported Consistency of findings: No, studies showed mixed results	Inconclusive; low	Included studies were not quality rated. Variability in outcome measures used and in the administration of SPT. Findings are based on small sample sizes.	Requires a master's level counselor for implementation.
Validation Therapy	3 RCTs and 2 other studies with small samples (N=5) in each	Most recent search date: March 2006 Follow-up: 6 weeks to 12 months Consistency in findings: No, studies showed mixed results.	Inconclusive; low	Small sample sizes.	Requires a master's level counselor for implementation. Included studies had high levels of intervention intensity.
Stimulation Oriented Approaches					
Acupuncture	No studies met inclusion criteria	Most recent search date: February 2007	Inconclusive; no studies	NA	Requires a certified therapist.
Aromatherapy	1 RCT and 1 other study	Most recent search date: March 2008 Follow-up: ≤ 4 weeks Consistency of findings: Yes	Positive effect on agitation; low	Findings are based on a small sample. Possible problems with heterogeneity and other confounding variables.	May be easily implemented in a group setting without extensive training.
Light Therapy	4 RCTs, 4 other studies	Most recent search date: December 2005 Follow-up: No follow-up to 1 week Consistency of findings: No, studies showed mixed results	Positive effects on agitation and sleep; low	Overall findings are based on a small number of poor quality studies with very small sample sizes.	Depends on the method of therapy administered.
Massage and Touch	3 RCTs	Most recent search date: July 2005 Follow-up: 1 hr post treatment to 5 days Consistency of findings: Yes	Positive effects on agitation; low	Study findings are based on small sample sizes and limited treatment duration. Similar to calming music in preventing agitation. Support for massage compared to no treatment.	Depends on the type of therapy: A licensed massage therapist would be needed for some treatments; hand massage and touch therapy may be easier to implement. The increased stimulus could increase agitation and aggression in some individuals.
Music Therapy	4 SRs that included 3 RCTs	Study designs: Mostly time series in which subjects served as their own controls; also RCTs and case studies Quality rating: RCTs were poor Data sparseness: Samples were small; the largest study had 39 subjects Consistency of findings: Yes	Positive effects on agitation; low	Limitations: Well-conducted studies are lacking. Benefits appear to be short-term.	Some music interventions are simple and low-cost (e.g., playing recorded music at mealtimes) and may be feasible for wide implementation. The increased stimulus could increase agitation and aggression in some individuals.

Non-pharmacological Interventions for Behavioral Symptoms of Dementia

Intervention	Studies included in Systematic Reviews (SRs)	Quality of data: Most recent search date Length of follow-up Consistency of findings	Estimate of benefit; overall level of evidence	Study limitations	Comments on feasibility and acceptability
Snoezelen Multisensory Therapy	6 RCTs	Most recent search date: March 2008 Follow-up: ≤ 1 month Consistency of findings: No, studies showed mixed results	Inconclusive; moderate	Variability of intervention components in included studies.	May be easily implemented in a group setting without extensive training.
Transcutaneous Electrical Nerve Stimulation (TENS)	3 RCTs	Most recent search date: December 2005 Follow-up: ≤ 6 weeks Consistency of findings: Yes (data were pooled)	Neutral effect; low	Individual studies consisted of small sample sizes.	Would most likely require a trained OT or PT or master's level psychologist.
Behavior Management Techniques					
Behavior Management Techniques	7 RCTs plus 2 recent primary studies identified by peer review	Most recent search date within SRs: January 2006 Follow-up: ≤ 9 months Consistency of findings: No, studies showed mixed results	Mixed results across outcomes; low	Inadequate blinding procedures; control groups primarily usual care rather than alternative interventions.	Varies based on type of intervention; many interventions likely able to be implemented in VA settings, though individualization to patients is often needed. Likely requires master's level therapist or psychologist.
Other Psychosocial Interventions					
Animal-assisted Therapy	9 primary studies, no RCTs	Study design: Uncontrolled time series and non-randomized controlled trials Quality rating: Not applicable to study design Data sparseness: # participants ranged from 6 to 62 per study/length of follow-up ranged from same day of intervention to 4 weeks Consistency of findings: No, studies showed mixed results	Positive effects on agitation, passivity, social interactions, and nutritional intake; very low	Studies were small and heterogeneous, and lacked methodological rigor.	Among the therapies studied, fish aquariums and visiting dog therapy may be feasible for broad implementation in VA.
Exercise	3 SRs: 18 RCTs and 17 other trials	Most recent search date: September 2007 Follow-up: 5 days to 24 months Consistency in findings: No, studies showed mixed results	Positive effects on sleep; very low overall; moderate for outcome of sleep	Small sample sizes, variation in intervention intensity and duration, variation in baseline dementia severity. Poor methodology.	Varies based on intensity of intervention, but some interventions (e.g., walking) could be accomplished without specialized training.

Intervention	Studies included in Systematic Reviews (SRs)	Quality of data: Most recent search date Length of follow-up Consistency of findings	Estimate of benefit; overall level of evidence	Study limitations	Comments on feasibility and acceptability
Targeted Behavioral Symptoms					
Wandering	Subjective barriers: No RCTs met inclusion criteria	Most recent search date: March 2009	NA; no evidence	NA	NA
	Various sensory stimulation therapies: 8 RCTs, 3 non-RCT parallel and cross-over studies	Most recent search date: October 2005 Follow-up: range 3 days to < 1 year (mean 6 weeks) Consistency of findings: No, studies showed mixed results	Inconclusive; low	Evidence is based on a small number of studies within each intervention category. Quality of studies was poor, with limited methodological reporting.	Music, exercise, and multisensory stimulation appear to be pleasant and enjoyable for patients. The increased stimulation could increase agitation and aggression in some individuals. These interventions are likely easy to implement in VA settings at low cost.
	GPS tracking devices, boundary alarms, other monitoring devices	Case studies; cross-sectional studies; or single-group, pre- and post-test/post-test only studies. Search date through 2006.	Improved patient safety; very low	Studies were small and lacked a control group.	Costly and resource intensive, requiring training and technical support. Increases caregiver peace of mind.
Agitation	7 RCTs and 7 randomized cross-over studies, plus 1 recent primary study identified by peer review	Follow-up: Up to 2 months (study grouped follow-up < 2 mos. and > 2 mos.) Consistency of findings: Yes (data were pooled)	Positive effects on agitation with sensory interventions and systematic individualized intervention; low	Small number of studies for each type of therapy; variability in duration of treatment and measuring instruments.	Aromatherapy, thermal bath, calming music, and hand massage are low-cost and have some evidence of benefit.
Inappropriate Sexual Behavior	No SRs found	There is no available evidence to support or refute the effectiveness of non-pharmacological treatments for inappropriate sexual behavioral among patients with dementia.	NA	NA	NA

41

REFERENCES

1. Veterans Health Administration Office of the Assistant Deputy Under Secretary for Health for Policy and Planning. Projections of the prevalence and incidence of dementias including Alzheimer's Disease for the total, enrolled, and patient veteran populations aged 65 or over. 2004. *http://www4.va.gov/HEALTHPOLICYPLANNING/reports1.asp*.

2. Teri L, Logsdon RG, McCurry SM. Nonpharmacologic treatment of behavioral disturbance in dementia. *Med Clin North Am.* 2002 May 2002;86(3):641-656.

3. Zetteler J. Effectiveness of simulated presence therapy for individuals with dementia: a systematic review and meta-analysis. *Aging Ment Health.* Nov 2008;12(6):779-785.

4. National Institute for Health and Clinical Excellence (NICE). Dementia: A NICE–SCIE Guideline on supporting people with dementia and their careers in health and social care. *National Clinical Practice Guideline Number 42.* Vol: The British Psychological Society and Gaskell; 2007.

5. Opie J, Rosewarne R, O'Connor DW. The efficacy of psychosocial approaches to behaviour disorders in dementia: a systematic literature review. *Aust N Z J Psychiatry.* Dec 1999;33(6):789-799.

6. McDonagh MS, Peterson K, Carson S, Chan B, Thakurta S. Drug class review on atypical antipsychotic drugs. Update #2 final report. *http://www.ohsu.edu/drugeffectiveness/reports/final.cfm*. 2009.

7. Ayalon L, Gum AM, Feliciano L, Arean PA. Effectiveness of nonpharmacological interventions for the management of neuropsychiatric symptoms in patients with dementia: a systematic review. *Arch Intern Med.* Nov 13 2006;166(20):2182-2188.

8. Goy E, Freeman M, Kansagara D. A systematic evidence review of interventions for non-professional caregivers of patients with dementia. A report by the Evidence-based Synthesis Program of Veterans Health Administration, Health Services Research & Development. Washington, DC. May, 2009.

9. Brozek JL, Akl EA, Alonso-Coello P, et al. Grading quality of evidence and strength of recommendations in clinical practice guidelines. Part 1 of 3. An overview of the GRADE approach and grading quality of evidence about interventions. *Allergy.* May 2009;64(5):669-677.

10. Woods B, Spector AE, Jones CA, Orrell M, Davies SP. Reminiscence therapy for dementia. *Cochrane Database of Systematic Reviews.* 2009(3).

11. Livingston G, Johnston K, Katona C, Paton J, Lyketsos CG, Old Age Task Force of the World Federation of Biological P. Systematic review of psychological approaches to the management of neuropsychiatric symptoms of dementia. *Am J Psychiatry.* Nov 2005;162(11):1996-2021.

12.   O'Connor DW, Ames D, Gardner B, King M. Psychosocial treatments of psychological symptoms in dementia: a systematic review of reports meeting quality standards. *Int Psychogeriatr.* Apr 2009;21(2):241-251.

13.   O'Connor DW, Ames D, Gardner B, King M. Psychosocial treatments of behavior symptoms in dementia: a systematic review of reports meeting quality standards. *Int Psychogeriatr.* Apr 2009;21(2):225-240.

14.   Neal M, Barton Wright P. Validation therapy for dementia. *Cochrane Database of Systematic Reviews.* 2009(3).

15.   Weina P, Zhao H, Zhishun L, Shi W. Acupuncture for vascular dementia. *Cochrane Database of Systematic Reviews.* 2009(2).

16.   Holt FE, Birks TPH, Thorgrimsen LM, Spector AE, Wiles A, Orrell M. Aroma therapy for dementia. *Cochrane Database of Systematic Reviews.* 2009(3).

17.   Forbes D, Morgan DG, Bangma J, Peacock S, Adamson J. Light Therapy for Managing Sleep, Behaviour, and Mood Disturbances in Dementia. *Cochrane Database of Systematic Reviews.* 2009(3).

18.   Hansen NV, Jorgensen T, Ortenblad L. Massage and touch for dementia. *Cochrane Database of Systematic Reviews.* 2009(3).

19.   Gleeson M, Timmins F. The use of touch to enhance nursing care of older person in long-term mental health care facilities. *Journal of Psychiatric & Mental Health Nursing.* Oct 2004;11(5):541-545.

20.   Cuddy LL, Duffin J, Cuddy LL, Duffin J. Music, memory, and Alzheimer's disease: is music recognition spared in dementia, and how can it be assessed? *Med Hypotheses.* 2005;64(2):229-235.

21.   Braben I. A Song for Mrs. Smith. *Nursing Times.* 1992;88(41):54.

22.   Swartz KP, Hantz EC, Crummer GC, Walton JP, Frisina RD. Does the melody linger on? Music cognition in Alzheimer's disease. *Semin Neurol.* Jun 1989;9(2):152-158.

23.   Brotons M, Koger SM, Pickett-Cooper P. Music and dementias: A review of literature. *Journal of Music Therapy.* Win 1997;34(4):204-245.

24.   Vink AC, Birks J, Bruinsma MS, Scholten RJPM. Music therapy for people with dementia. *Cochrane Database of Systematic Reviews.* 2009(3).

25.   Sung HC, Chang AM. Use of preferred music to decrease agitated behaviours in older people with dementia: a review of the literature. *J Clin Nurs.* Oct 2005;14(9):1133-1140.

26.   Sherratt K, Thornton A, Hatton C. Music interventions for people with dementia: A review of the literature. *Aging & Mental Health.* Jan 2004;8(1):3-12.

27.   Clark ME, Lipe AW, Bilbrey M. Use of music to decrease aggressive behaviors in people with dementia. *J Gerontol Nurs.* Jul 1998;24(7):10-17.

28.   Gerdner LA. Effects of individualized versus classical "relaxation" music on the frequency of agitation in elderly persons with Alzheimer's disease and related disorders. *International Psychogeriatrics*. Mar 2000;12(1):49-65.

29.   Groene RW. Effectiveness of music therapy 1:1 intervention with individuals having senile dementia of the Alzheimer's type. *Journal of Music Therapy*. 1993;30(3):138-157.

30.   Ragneskog H, Brane G, Karlsson I, Kihlgren M. Influence of dinner music on food intake and symptoms common in dementia. *Scand J Caring Sci*. 1996;10(1):11-17.

31.   Chung JCC, Lai CKY. Snoezelen for dementia. *Cochrane Database of Systematic Reviews*. 2009(3).

32.   Verkaik R, van Weert JC, Francke AL. The effects of psychosocial methods on depressed, aggressive and apathetic behaviors of people with dementia: a systematic review. *Int J Geriatr Psychiatry*. Apr 2005;20(4):301-314.

33.   Johnson MI. *Electrotherapy: Evidence-Based Practice*: Ed. Watson. T. Elsevier; 2008.

34.   Cameron MH, Lonergan E, Lee H. Transcutaneous Electrical Nerve Stimulation (TENS) for dementia. *Cochrane Database of Systematic Reviews*. 2009(3).

35.   Logsdon RG, McCurry SM, Teri L. Evidence-based psychological treatments for disruptive behaviors in individuals with dementia. *Psychol Aging*. Vol 22. 2007/03/28 ed. 2007:28-36.

36.   Proctor R, Burns A, Powell HS, et al. Behavioural management in nursing and residential homes: a randomised controlled trial. *Lancet*. Jul 3 1999;354(9172):26-29.

37.   Teri L, Gibbons LE, McCurry SM, et al. Exercise plus behavioral management in patients with Alzheimer disease: a randomized controlled trial. *JAMA*. Oct 15 2003;290(15):2015-2022.

38.   Teri L, McCurry SM, Logsdon R, et al. Training community consultants to help family members improve dementia care: a randomized controlled trial. *Gerontologist*. Dec 2005;45(6):802-811.

39.   Teri L, Huda P, Gibbons L, et al. STAR: a dementia-specific training program for staff in assisted living residences. *Gerontologist*. Oct 2005;45(5):686-693.

40.   Gitlin LN, Winter L, Dennis MP, et al. A biobehavioral home-based intervention and the well-being of patients with dementia and their caregivers: the COPE randomized trial. *JAMA*. Sep 1 2010;304(9):983-991.

41.   Beck CK, Vogelpohl TS, Rasin JH, et al. Effects of behavioral interventions on disruptive behavior and affect in demented nursing home residents. *Nurs Res*. Jul-Aug 2002;51(4):219-228.

42.   Suhr J, Anderson S, Tranel D. Progressive Muscle Relaxation in theManagement of Behavioural Disturbance in Alzheimer's Disease. *Neuropsychological Rehabilitation.* 1999;9(1):31-44.

43.   McCallion P, Toseland RW, Freeman K. An evaluation of a family visit education program. *J Am Geriatr Soc.* Feb 1999;47(2):203-214.

44.   Teri L, Logsdon RG, Uomoto J, McCurry SM. Behavioral treatment of depression in dementia patients: a controlled clinical trial. *J Gerontol B Psychol Sci Soc Sci.* Jul 1997;52(4):P159-166.

45.   Teri LP, Gibbons LEP, McCurry SMP, et al. Exercise Plus Behavioral Management in Patients With Alzheimer Disease: A Randomized Controlled Trial. *JAMA.* 2003;290(15):2015-2022.

46.   Centre for Evidence Based Medicine. Levels of Evidence (March 2009). *http://www. cebm.net/index.aspx?o=1025* Accessed Feb. 15, 2011.

47.   Libin A, Cohen-Mansfield J. Therapeutic robocat for nursing home residents with dementia: preliminary inquiry. *Am J Alzheimers Dis Other Demen.* Mar-Apr 2004;19(2):111-116.

48.   Greer KL, Pustay KA, Zaun TC, Coppens P. A comparison of the effects of toys versus live animals on the communication of patients with dementia of the Alzheimer's type. *Clinical Gerontologist: The Journal of Aging and Mental Health.* 2001;24(3-4):157-182.

49.   Martindale BP. Effect of animal-assisted therapy on engagement of rural nursing home residents. *American Journal of Recreation Therapy.* 2008;7(4):45-53.

50.   McCabe BW, Baun MM, Speich D, Agrawal S. Resident dog in the Alzheimer's special care unit. *West J Nurs Res.* Oct 2002;24(6):684-696.

51.   Edwards NE, Beck AM. Animal-assisted therapy and Nutrition in Alzheimer's disease. *West J Nurs Res.* Oct 2002;24(6):697-712.

52.   Richeson NE. Effects of animal-assisted therapy on agitated behaviors and social interactions of older adults with dementia. *Am J Alzheimers Dis Other Demen.* Nov-Dec 2003;18(6):353-358.

53.   Churchill M, Safaoui J, McCabe BW, Baun MM. Using a therapy dog to alleviate the agitation and desocialization of people with Alzheimer's disease. *J Psychosoc Nurs Ment Health Serv.* Apr 1999;37(4):16-22.

54.   Batson K, McCabe B, Baun MM, Wilson C. *The effect of a therapy dog on socialization and physiological indicators of stress in persons diagnosed with Alzheimer's disease.* Thousand Oaks, CA: Sage Publications, Inc; 1998.

55.   Kongable LG, Buckwalter KC, Stolley JM. The effects of pet therapy on the social behavior of institutionalized Alzheimer's clients. *Arch Psychiatr Nurs.* Aug 1989;3(4):191-198.

56. Forbes D, Forbes S, Morgan DG, Markle-Reid M, Wood J, Culum I. Physical activity programs for persons with dementia. *Cochrane Database of Systematic Reviews.* 2009(3).

57. Eggermont LH, Scherder EJ. Physical activity and behaviour in dementia: A review of the literature and implications for psychosocial intervention in primary care. *Dementia: The International Journal of Social Research and Practice.* Aug 2006;5(3):411-428.

58. Heyn P, Abreu BC, Ottenbacher KJ. The effects of exercise training on elderly persons with cognitive impairment and dementia: a meta-analysis. *Arch Phys Med Rehabil.* Oct 2004;85(10):1694-1704.

59. Holliman DC, Orgassa UC, Forney JP. Developing an interactive physical activity group in a geriatric psychiatry facility. *Activities, Adaptation and Aging.* 2001;26(1):57-69.

60. Rolland Y, Pillard F, Klapouszczak A, et al. Exercise program for nursing home residents with Alzheimer's disease: a 1-year randomized, controlled trial. *J Am Geriatr Soc.* Feb 2007;55(2):158-165.

61. Stevens J, Killeen M, Stevens J, Killeen M. A randomised controlled trial testing the impact of exercise on cognitive symptoms and disability of residents with dementia. *Contemp Nurse.* Feb-Mar 2006;21(1):32-40.

62. Francese T, Sorrell J, Butler FR. The effects of regular exercise on muscle strength and functional abilities of late stage Alzheimer's residents. *American Journal of Alzheimer's Disease and Other Dementias.* 1997;12(3):122-127.

63. Alessi CA, Yoon EJ, Schnelle JF, Al-Samarrai NR, Cruise PA. A randomized trial of a combined physical activity and environmental intervention in nursing home residents: do sleep and agitation improve? *J Am Geriatr Soc.* Jul 1999;47(7):784-791.

64. McCurry SM, Gibbons LE, Logsdon RG, et al. Nighttime insomnia treatment and education for Alzheimer's disease: a randomized, controlled trial. *J Am Geriatr Soc.* May 2005;53(5):793-802.

65. Mulrow CD, Gerety MB, Kanten D, et al. A randomized trial of physical rehabilitation for very frail nursing home residents. *JAMA.* Feb 16 1994;271(7):519-524.

66. Van de Winckel A, Feys H, De Weerdt W, et al. Cognitive and behavioural effects of music-based exercises in patients with dementia. *Clinical Rehabilitation.* May 2004;18(3):253-260.

67. Alessi CA, Martin JL, Webber AP, et al. Randomized, controlled trial of a nonpharmacological intervention to improve abnormal sleep/wake patterns in nursing home residents. *J Am Geriatr Soc.* May 2005;53(5):803-810.

68. Baum EE, Jarjoura D, Polen AE, et al. Effectiveness of a group exercise program in a long-term care facility: a randomized pilot trial. *Journal of the American Medical Directors Association.* Mar-Apr 2003;4(2):74-80.

69.   Hermans D, Htay UH, McShane R. Non-pharmacological interventions for wandering of people with dementia in the domestic setting. *Cochrane Database of Systematic Reviews.* 2009(3).

70.   Price JD, Hermans D, Grimley Evans J. Subjective barriers to prevent wandering of cognitively impaired people. *Cochrane Database of Systematic Reviews.* 2009(3).

71.   Robinson L, Hutchings D, Corner L, et al. A systematic literature review of the effectiveness of non-pharmacological interventions to prevent wandering in dementia and evaluation of the ethical implications and acceptability of their use. *Health Technol Assess.* Aug 2006;10(26):iii, ix-108.

72.   Robinson L, Hutchings D, Dickinson HO, et al. Effectiveness and acceptability of non-pharmacological interventions to reduce wandering in dementia: a systematic review. *Int J Geriatr Psychiatry.* Jan 2007;22(1):9-22.

73.   Lauriks S, Reinersmann A, Van der Roest HG, et al. Review of ICT-based services for identified unmet needs in people with dementia. *Ageing Res Rev.* Oct 2007;6(3):223-246.

74.   Kong EH, Evans LK, Guevara JP. Nonpharmacological intervention for agitation in dementia: a systematic review and meta-analysis. *Aging Ment Health.* Jul 2009;13(4):512-520.

75.   Cohen-Mansfield J, Libin A, Marx MS. Nonpharmacological treatment of agitation: a controlled trial of systematic individualized intervention. *J Gerontol A Biol Sci Med Sci.* Aug 2007;62(8):908-916.

76.   Luijpen MW, Scherder EJ, Van Someren EJ, Swaab DF, Sergeant JA. Non-pharmacological interventions in cognitively impaired and demented patients--a comparison with cholinesterase inhibitors. *Rev Neurosci.* 2003;14(4):343-368.

77.   American Veterinary Medical Association. Guidelines for Animal Assisted Activity, Animal-Assisted Therapy and Resident Animal Programs. *Current as of 2007.* *http://www.avma.org/issues/policy/animal_assisted_guidelines.asp.*

78.   Henderson NK, White CP, Eisman JA. The roles of exercise and fall risk reduction in the prevention of osteoporosis. *Endocrinol Metab Clin North Am.* Jun 1998;27(2):369-387.

79.   Carter ND, Kannus P, Khan KM. Exercise in the prevention of falls in older people: a systematic literature review examining the rationale and the evidence. *Sports Med.* 2001;31(6):427-438.

80.   Inouye SK, Bogardus ST, Jr., Charpentier PA, et al. A multicomponent intervention to prevent delirium in hospitalized older patients. *N Engl J Med.* Mar 4 1999;340(9):669-676.

81.   Atkins D, Best D, Briss PA, et al. Grading quality of evidence and strength of recommendations. *Bmj.* Jun 19 2004;328(7454):1490.

APPENDIX A. SEARCH STRATEGY FOR NON-PHARMACO-LOGICAL TREATMENT OF DEMENTIA, REVIEWS

MEDLINE (PubMed) searched on 10/08/2009

Search #	Concept	Search String	N
1	Dementia	"dementia"[MeSH Terms] OR "dementia"[All Fields] OR dement*[tiab] OR "mild cognitive impairment" [tiab]	110,737
2	Non-Pharmacological treatments	("non pharmacologic*"[tiab] OR "non-pharmacologic*"[tiab] OR "nonpharmacologic*"[tiab]) AND (therapy [tiab] OR intervention [tiab])	1,357
3	Psychotherapy	"psychotherapy"[MeSH Terms] OR "psychotherapy"[tiab]	126,941
4	exercise/physical activity	"Exercise/therapy"[Mesh] OR "Exercise Therapy"[Mesh] OR "exercise"[tiab] OR "motor activity"[MeSH Terms] OR ("motor"[tiab] AND "activity"[tiab]) OR "motor activity"[tiab] OR ("physical"[tiab] AND "activity"[tiab]) OR "physical activity"[tiab]	281,156
5	transcutaneous electrical nerve stimulation (TENS)	"transcutaneous electrical nerve stimulation"[tiab] OR ("transcutaneous electric nerve stimulation"[MeSH Terms] OR ("transcutaneous"[tiab] AND "electric"[tiab] AND "nerve"[tiab] AND "stimulation"[tiab]) OR "tens"[tiab])	9,317
6	snoezelen multi-sensory stimulation	"Snoezelen" OR "multisensory stimulation" OR "multi sensory stimulation" OR "multi-sensory stimulation" OR "multisensory environment" OR "multi sensory environment" OR "multi-sensory environment"	108
7	bright light therapy	"phototherapy"[MeSH Terms] OR "phototherapy"[tiab] OR ("light"[tiab] AND "therapy"[tiab]) OR "light therapy"[tiab] OR "photo-therapy"[tiab] OR "light-therapy"[tiab]	31,862
8	smart home technologies	(Home-based[tiab] AND (assistive technologies[tiab] OR assistive technology[tiab])) OR smart home technologies[tiab] OR smart home technology[tiab] OR ("Telemetry"[Mesh] OR "Telemedicine"[Mesh])	16,073
9	acupuncture	"acupuncture"[MeSH Terms] OR "acupuncture"[tiab] OR "acupuncture therapy"[MeSH Terms]	14,240
10	massage and touch therapies	("touch"[MeSH Terms] OR "touch"[tiab]) AND ("therapy"[Subheading] OR "therapy"[tiab] OR "therapeutics"[MeSH Terms] OR "therapeutics"[tiab]) OR "Massage"[Mesh] OR "massage" [tiab]	13,184
11	music therapy	"music therapy"[MeSH Terms] OR ("music"[tiab] AND "therapy"[tiab]) OR "music therapy"[tiab]	1,990
12	sensory stimulation	"sensory stimulation"[tiab]	1,514
13	aromatherapy	"aromatherapy"[MeSH Terms] OR "aromatherapy"[tiab] OR ("aroma"[tiab] AND "therapy"[tiab]) OR "aroma therapy"[tiab]	590
14	reality orientation	"Reality Therapy"[Mesh] OR reality orientation [tiab] OR reality therapy [tiab]	374
15	behavioral management	(behavior* [tiab] AND management [tiab]) OR Behavior Therapy [MeSH]	50,249
16	simulated presence	"simulated presence" [tiab]	10
17	reminiscence therapy	("reminisce" [tiab] OR "reminiscence" [tiab]) AND ("therapy" [tiab] OR "technique*" [tiab] OR "treatment" [tiab] OR "intervention" [tiab] OR "group" [tiab])	224
18	validation therapy	"validation" [tiab] AND ("therapy" [tiab] OR "technique*" [tiab] OR "treatment" [tiab] OR "intervention" [tiab])	13,769

19	all treatments	OR (#2-18)	506,887
20	all treatments for dementia	#19 AND #1	4,729
21	non-indexed articles from set #20	#20 AND (in process[sb] OR publisher[sb] OR pubmednotmedline[sb])	140
22	indexed articles from set #20	#20 NOT #21	4,589
23	articles indexed as systematic reviews	#22 AND systematic [sb]	196
24	(systematic reviews, or un-indexed) English only	(#23 OR #21) AND English[lang]	304

The symptoms, comparators, outcomes and settings are best dealt with using inclusion and exclusion criteria, including them in the search risks artificially limiting the search results.

PsycINFO (OVID)searched on 10/08/2009			
Search #	**Concept**	**Search String**	**N**
1	Dementia	exp dementia/ or exp alzheimers disease/ or exp cognitive impairment/ or Dementia.mp.	52,506
2	Psychotherapy	psychotherapy.mp. or exp Psychotherapy/	169,679
3	exercise/physical activity	exp physical activity/ or exercise.mp. or physical activity.mp.	30,661
4	transcutaneous electrical nerve stimulation (TENS)	exp Electrical Stimulation/ or transcutaneous electrical nerve stimulation.mp. or tens.mp.	14,847
5	snoezelen multi-sensory stimulation	snoezelen.mp. or perceptual stimulation.mp. or exp Perceptual Stimulation/ or multi sensory stimulation.mp. or multi sensory environment.mp.	49,928
6	bright light therapy	light therapy.mp. or exp Phototherapy/	801
7	smart home technologies	(exp Technology/ and exp Housing/) or smart home.mp. or exp telemedicine/	1,122
8	acupuncture	acupuncture.mp. or exp Acupuncture/	759
9	massage and touch therapies	exp Massage/ or massage.mp. or exp Physical Contact/ or touch therapy.mp.	2,162
10	music therapy	music therapy.mp. or exp Music Therapy/	2,763
11	aromatherapy	aromatherapy/ or olfactory stimulation/ or (aromatherapy or aroma therapy).mp.	1,1661
12	reality orientation	exp Reality Therapy/ or reality orientation.mp. or reality therapy.mp.	964
13	behavioral management	exp Behavior Therapy/ or exp Behavior Modification/ or behavioral management.mp.	34,227
14	simulated presence	simulated presence.mp.	12
15	reminiscence therapy	exp Reminiscence/ or reminiscence therapy.mp.	1,200
16	validation therapy	validation therapy.mp.	39
17	all treatments	OR (#2-16)	286,924
18	all treatments for dementia	#17 AND #1	2.150
19	systematic reviews	limit #18 to ("0800 literature review" or "0830 systematic review" or 1200 meta analysis)	127
20	English	limit 19 to english language	120
After de-duplication with PubMed results : 102 unique citations			

Cochrane Database of Systematic Reviews & Cochrane Database of Abstracts of Reviews of Effects (OVID) searched on 10/08/2009

Search #	Concept	Search String	N
1	Dementia	dementia.mp. or alzheimers.mp. or cognitive impairment.mp.	559
2	Non-Pharmacological treatments	non-pharmacological treatment.mp.	37
3	Psychotherapy	Psychotherapy.mp.	587
4	exercise/physical activity	exercise.mp. or physical activity.mp.	1,750
5	transcutaneous electrical nerve stimulation (TENS)	transcutaneous electrical nerve stimulation.mp. or tens.mp.	181
6	snoezelen multi-sensory stimulation	snoezelen.mp. or multi sensory environment.mp. or multi-sensory stimulation.mp.	10
7	bright light therapy	light therapy.mp. or phototherapy.mp.	0
8	smart home technologies	smart home.mp. or telemedicine.mp.	60
9	acupuncture	acupuncture.mp.	1
10	massage and touch therapies	massage.mp. or touch.mp.	391
11	music therapy	music therapy.mp.	78
12	sensory stimulation	sensory stimulation.mp.	23
13	aromatherapy	(aromatherapy or aroma therapy).mp.	45
14	reality orientation	reality orientation.mp. or reality therapy.mp.	18
15	behavioral management	behavioral management.mp. or behavior therapy.mp. or behavior modification.mp.	270
16	simulated presence	simulated presence.mp.	6
17	reminiscence therapy	reminiscence therapy.mp.	11
18	validation therapy	validation therapy.mp.	5
19	all treatments	OR (#2-18)	2,848
20	all treatments for dementia	#19 AND #1	158

No duplicated detected by EndNote

APPENDIX B. SEARCH STRATEGY FOR PRIMARY STUDIES ON ANIMAL-ASSISTED THERAPY FOR DEMENTIA

PubMed search 12/9/2009, 275 results

"humans"[MeSH Terms] AND (((((((((((pet therapy[tiab] OR animal assisted therapy[tiab]) OR animal therapy[tiab]) OR dog therapy[tiab]) OR dog assisted therapy[tiab]) OR animal-assisted activities[tiab]) OR animal-assisted interventions[tiab]) OR aquarium[tiab]) OR (("Dogs"[Mesh] OR "Cats"[Mesh]) OR "Birds"[Mesh])) OR ("Bonding, Human-Pet"[Mesh] OR "Animals, Domestic"[Mesh])) AND ("dementia"[MeSH Terms] OR "dementia"[All Fields]))

PsycINFO search 12/9/2009, 83 results (61 unique)

PsycINFO 1806 to December Week 2 2009

#	Searches	Results
1	pet therapy.mp. or exp Animal Assisted Therapy/	335
2	animal assisted therapy.mp. or exp Animal Assisted Therapy/	330
3	animal assisted therapy.mp.	330
4	exp Interspecies Interaction/ or exp Pets/ or exp Dogs/	5351
5	dog therapy.mp.	8
6	dog assisted therapy.mp.	3
7	animal assisted activities.mp.	18
8	animal assisted interventions.mp.	10
9	aquarium.mp.	269
10	cats.mp. or exp Cats/	11113
11	birds.mp. or exp Birds/	22735
12	1 or 2 or 3 or 4 or 5 or 6 or 7 or 8 or 9 or 10 or 11	38995
13	dementia.mp. or exp Dementia/	45487
14	12 and 13	83
15	from 14 keep 1-10	10
16	from 14 keep 1-83	83

CINAHL search 12/9/2009, 65 results (44 unique)

#	Searches	Results
S14	S12 and S13	65
S13	("dementia") or (MH "Dementia+")	23,299
S12	S1 or S2 or S3 or S4 or S5 or S6 or S7 or S8 or S9 or S10 or S11	3,595
S11	("birds") or (MH "Birds")	926
S10	("cats") or (MH "Cats")	923
S9	aquarium	20
S8	"animal assisted interventions"	7
S7	"animal assisted activities"	4
S6	("dog assisted therapy") or (MH "Service Animals")	126
S5	"dog therapy"	0
S4	("pets") or (MH "Pets")	1,279
S3	("human pet bonding") or (MH "Human-Pet Bonding")	288
S2	"animal assisted therapy"	105
S1	("pet therapy") or (MH "Pet Therapy")	526

Deduplication notes – MPF 10Dec09
Total citations after deduplication = 371

APPENDIX C. INCLUSION/EXCLUSION CRITERIA FOR SYSTEMATIC REVIEWS OF NON-PHARMACOLOGICAL INTERVENTIONS

1. Is the publication a systematic review/meta-analysis of clinical trials or observational studies?
   a. No ....STOP ☐
   b. Yes .... ☐

2. Does the study population at least partly include patients with dementia?
   a. No ....STOP ☐
   b. Yes .... ☐

3. Was the study conducted in an outpatient care setting (including home-based care, ambulatory care, and extended-care facilities)?
   a. No ....STOP ☐
   b. Yes .... ☐

4. Does the study address the following behavioral symptoms: apathy, agitation, disturbed sleep, wandering, impulsivity, disinhibition, depression, or inappropriate sexual behavior?
   a. No ....STOP ☐
   b. Yes .... ☐

5. Does the study evaluate the effectiveness, safety, or cost of any of the following types of interventions?
   Acupuncture .... ☐
   Animal-assisted therapy .... ☐
   Aromatherapy .... ☐
   Exercise / physical activity .... ☐
   Light therapy .... ☐
   Massage and touch therapies .... ☐
   Music Therapy .... ☐
   Psychotherapy; e.g., behavioral mgmt, cognitive stimulation or rehabilitation, reality orientation, simulated presence, reminiscence, validation .... ☐
   Snoezelen or other sensory stimulation .... ☐
   Smart home technologies: (social alarms, electronic assistive devices, environmental control systems, automated home environments) .... ☐
   Transcutaneous Electrical Nerve Stimulation (TENS) .... ☐
   Other, non-pharmacological treatment, specify .... ☐
   None of the above ....STOP

6. Does the comparator intervention consist of any of the following: another non-pharmacological treatment, medical/ pharmacological treatment, or no treatment? Note: ECT is considered medical treatment.
   a. No ....STOP ☐
   b. Yes .... ☐

7. Does the study report on any of the following patient outcomes?
   Use of psychotropic drugs .... ☐
   Cognition .... ☐
   Mood .... ☐
   Behavioral disturbances .... ☐
   Social function .... ☐
   Physical function .... ☐
   Hospitalizations, institutionalization, or other healthcare visits, including; ER visits .... ☐
   Accidents .... ☐
   Health-related quality of life .... ☐
   Satisfaction with healthcare .... ☐
   Other, specify .... ☐
   None of the above ....Proceed to Q8

8. Is the text of the article in English?
   a. No ....STOP ☐
   b. Yes .... ☐

9. If this article meets no other criterion, should it be saved for background or discussion?
   a. No ....STOP ☐
   b. Yes: narrative review with potentially useful references .... ☐
   c. Yes: primary study, possibly more recent than existing SRs .... ☐
   d. Yes: clinical guidelines .... ☐
   e. Yes: discusses methodological issues .... ☐
   f. Yes: systematic review that did not meet all quality criteria .... ☐

APPENDIX D. QUALITY RATING CRITERIA FOR SYSTEMATIC REVIEWS*

Overall quality rating for each systematic review is based on the below questions. Ratings are summarized as: *Good, Fair, or Poor*:

- Search dates reported? *Yes or No*
- Search methods reported? *Yes or No*
- Comprehensive search? *Yes or No*
- Inclusion criteria reported? *Yes or No*
- Selection bias avoided? *Yes or No*
- Validity criteria reported? *Yes or No*
- Validity assessed appropriately? *Yes or No*
- Methods used to combine studies reported? *Yes or No*
- Findings combined appropriately? *Yes or No*
- Conclusions supported by data? *Yes or No*

Definitions of ratings based on above criteria

Good: Meet all criteria: Reports comprehensive and reproducible search methods and results; reports pre-defined criteria to select studies, and reports reasons for excluding potentially relevant studies; adequately evaluates quality of included studies and incorporates assessments of quality when synthesizing data; reports methods for synthesizing data and uses appropriate methods to combine data qualitatively or quantitatively; conclusions supported by the evidence reviewed.

Fair: Studies will be graded fair if they fail to meet one or more of the above criteria, but the limitations are not judged as being major.

Poor: Studies will be graded poor if they have a major limitation in one or more of the above criteria.

*Created from the following publications:

Harris RP, Helfand M, Woolf SH, et al. Current methods of the US Preventive Services Task Force: a review of the process. *Am J Prev Med.* 2001:20(3S); 21-35.

National Institute for Health and Clinical Excellence. The Guidelines Manual. London: Institute for Health and Clinical Excellence; 2006.

Oxman AD, Guyatt GH. Validation of an index of the quality of review articles. *J Clin Epidemiol.* 1991;44:1271-8.

APPENDIX E. INCLUSION/EXCLUSION CRITERIA FOR PET/ANIMAL-ASSISTED THERAPY

1. Is the publication considered a controlled clinical trial?
   a. No...STOP ☐
   b. Yes (with control group) ....☐
      If yes, list study type:
      _____

2. Does the study population at least partly include patients with dementia?
   a. No...STOP ☐
   b. Yes...☐

3. Was the study conducted in an outpatient care setting (including home-based care, ambulatory care, and extended-care facilities)?
   a. No...STOP ☐
   b. Yes...☐

4. Does the study address any of the following behavioral symptoms: apathy, agitation, disruptive vocalizations, aggression, disturbed sleep, wandering, impulsivity, disinhibition, depression, inappropriate sexual behavior, or chronic/intermittent hallucinations and delusions?
   a. No...STOP ☐
   b. Yes...☐

5. Does the study evaluate the effectiveness, safety, or cost of any form of animal (pet) assisted therapy?
   a. No...STOP ☐
   b. Yes...☐

6. Does the comparator group consist of usual care (no treatment/intervention)?
   a. No...STOP ☐
   b. Yes...☐

7. Does the study report on any of the following patient outcomes?
   Use of psychotropic drugs...☐
   Cognition...☐
   Mood ....☐
   Behavioral disturbances ....☐
   Social function...☐
   Physical function...☐
   Hospitalizations, institutionalization, ER or other healthcare visits .....☐
   Accidents...☐
   Health-related quality of life ....☐
   Satisfaction with healthcare ....☐
   All cause mortality ....☐
   Other, specify..☐
   None of the above ....proceed to Q8

8. Is the text of the article in English?
   a. Yes...☒

9. If this article meets no other criterion, should it be saved for background, discussion, or other reasons?
   a. No...STOP
   b. Yes: narrative review, general description, reports of uncontrolled studies, informal observational studies with potentially useful references ....☐
   c. Yes: clinical guidelines...☐
   d. Yes: discusses methodological issues ....☐
   e. Yes: other non-pharmacological therapy, may apply to larger report....☐

APPENDIX F. ABBREVIATIONS

AA	African American
AARS	Apparent affect rating scale
AAT	Animal-assisted therapy
ABID	Agitated Behaviors in Dementia
AD	Alzheimer's disease
ADL	Activities of daily living
ADRDA	Alzheimer Disease and Related Disorders Association
AGECAT Organic, Depression	AGECAT is a computerised diagnostic system designed for use with the Geriatric Mental State and the History and Aetiology Schedule (designed to collect information about the history of the respondent with special reference to psychiatric illness including dementia, and about putative aetiological factors) for use in research with older people. AGECAT contains syndrome clusters for organic, anxiety, depression, etc.
AHRQ	Agency for Healthcare Research and Quality
AoA	Administration on Aging
BACS	Beliefs about Caregiving Scale
BAI	Beck Anxiety Inventory
BDI	Beck Depression Inventory
BDRS	Blessed Dementia Rating Scale
BEHAVE	Behavioral Pathology in Alzheimer's Disease Rating Scale
BMT	Behavior management training
BPRS	Brief Psychiatric Rating Scale
BRAD	Behavior Rating in AD
BVRT	Benton Visual Retention Test
CAS	Clinical Anxiety Scale
CES-D	Center for Epidemiologic Studies Depression Scale
CF	Category fluency
CG	Caregiver
CHS-M	Modified Caregiver Hassles Scale
CI	Confidence interval
CMAI-O, CMAI-N	Cohen-Mansfield Agitation Inventory - observer-derived score, nursing staff-derived score
COPE	Care of Persons with Dementia in their Environments
COWA	Controlled oral word association
CQLI	Caregiver Quality of Life Instrument
CR	Care recipient
CSDD	Cornell Scale for Depression in Dementia
CSQ	Caregiver sleep questionnaire
CTIS	Computer-Telephone Integration System
DBS	Disruptive behavior scale
DMSS	Dementia Management Strategies Scale
DRS	Depression Rating Scale
DSC	Dementia Steering Committee
ECR	Elderly Caregiver Family Relationship
EPC	Evidence Based Practice Center
ESP	Evidence-based Synthesis Program
FIM	Functional Independence Measure
GDRS	Geriatric Depression Rating Scale
GDS	Global Deterioration Scale
GIPB	Geriatric Indices of Positive Behavior
GPS	Global Positioning System
GQ-SRs	Good quality systematic reviews
HBPC	Home Based Primary Care
HDLF	Health and Daily Living Form
HDRS	Hamilton Depression Rating Scale
HSR&D	Health Services Research and Development
HTA	Health Technology Assessment
IADL	Instrumental Activities of Daily Living scale
ICT	Information and Communication Technology
ITT	Intention-to-treat
LSIZ	Life Satisfaction Index
LSNI	Lubben Social Network Index
LTC	Long-term care

Non-pharmacological Interventions for Behavioral Symptoms of Dementia

MAACL	Multiple Affect Adjective Checklist
MADDE	Medicare Alzheimer's Disease Demonstration and Evaluation program
MAI	Multilevel Assessment Inventory
MBPC	Memory and Behavior Problems Checklist
MFW	Minnesota Family Workshop
MMSE	Mini Mental State Exam
MOSES	Multidimensional Observation Scale for Older Subjects
MPB	Management of Problem Behaviors
MSS	Multisensory stimulation
N	Number
NHS	National Health Service
NIA/NINR	National Institute on Aging/National Institute of Nursing Research
NICE	National Institute for Health and Clinical Excellence
NINCDS	National Institute of Neurological and Communicative Diseases and Stroke
NPI	Neuropsychiatric Inventory
NYU	New York University
OARS	Older Americans Resource and Services Multidimensional Functional Assessment Questionnaire
ODAS	Observable displays of affect scale
OGEC	Office of Geriatrics and Extended Care
PAC	Positive Aspects of Caregiving scale
PAIS	Psychological Adjustment to Relative's Illness
PAVeD	Preventing Aggressive Behavior in Demented Patients
PCI	Patient Care Index
PDC	Partners in Dementia Care
PHQ9	Patient Health Questionnaire-9 Item
PIC	Partners in Caregiving
POMS	Profile of Moods States
PSS	Perceived Stress Scale
QALY	Quality of adjusted life years
QOL/QoL	Quality of life

RAGE	Rating Scale for Aggressive Behavior in the Elderly
RCT	Randomized controlled trial
REACH	Resources for Enhancing Alzheimer's Caregiver Health
RIL	Record of Independent Living
RMBPC	Revised Memory and Behavior Problem Checklist
RSCSE	Revised Scale for Caregiving Self-Efficacy
SADS	Social Avoidance and Distress Scale
SBP	Stress-Busting Program
SCB	Screen for Caregiver Burden
SCN	Suprachiasmatic nuclei
SF-36 (PF, PRF)	Short-form health survey (physical functioning and physical role functioning subscales)
SIP (BCM, M, HM)	Sickness Impact Profile (mobility scale; home management subscale
SPT	Simulated presence therapy
SR	Systematic Review
SSCQ	Short Sense of Competence Questionnaire
STAI	State Trait Anxiety Inventory
STAXI	State Trait Anger Expression Inventory
T1	Timepoint 1
T2	Timepoint 2
TENS	Transcutaneous electrical nerve stimulation
TLC	Telephone-Linked Care
Tx	Treatment
UK	United Kingdom
VA	Veterans Affairs
VAMC	Veterans Affairs Medical Center
VAS	Visual analog scale
VHA	Veterans Health Administration
VISN	Veterans Integrated Service Network
VSO	Visit Satisfaction Questionnaire
ZBI	Zarit Burden Interview

APPENDIX G. REVIEWER COMMENTS AND RESPONSES

Reviewer	Comment	Response
\multicolumn{3}{l}{**Are the objectives, scope, and methods for this review clearly described?**}		
1	Yes; no comment.	Noted.
2	Yes; no comment.	Noted.
3	Yes. The data is carefully addressed. An unfortunate feature of the study is that the results are largely negative. In spite of this, the findings are useful in determining appropriate care for people with dementia.	Noted.
4	P. 2: Several non-pharmacological interventions classified as "psychotherapy" (e.g., cognitive stimulation therapy, simulation presence therapy, and many behavioral management techniques) are not typically considered as psychotherapy. Furthermore, "behavior therapy" is referenced in the results and conclusion but is not listed as an intervention in the Methods section. It is also not clear what is meant by behavior therapy in the report. Additional specification or definition would be helpful, as this is often used broadly but technically involves a specific type of psychotherapy.	This section has been changed to clarify terminology and follow the outline of the report.
4	P. 3: The fact that the review included studies on management of behavioral symptoms of dementia in a wide variety of settings, including all outpatient settings, home-based care, and extended care settings may have affected the findings and contributed to mixed or non-conclusive results in some cases if data were analyzed in the aggregate. Certain interventions may work differently or require adaptation in different settings. It would be best to review and report results for different settings separately. This would also be helpful for guiding application of the results and future research directions.	There were insufficient numbers of behavior management studies to examine effects within subgroups by setting, provider type, and patient population, and therefore results were aggregated. The diversity of the settings examined across studies prohibited grouping based on this variable. Additionally, all behavior management technique studies had methodological limitations, and no subgroup of studies was exempt from these limitations.
\multicolumn{3}{l}{**Is there any indication of bias in our synthesis of the evidence?**}		
1	No; no comment.	Noted.
2	No; no comment.	Noted.
3	No; no comment.	Noted.
4	No; no comment.	Noted.
5	On search strategy - I do not see evidence of bias but am unclear as to whether there were search of primary studies that conducted on a particular topic between the time of the published systematic review and July 2009. Many of the systematic reviews in the Reference list were published in 2008 and 2009 but there are also several that were published before 2007. For those systematic reviews published prior to 2007, was a search conducted for more recent articles?	The breadth of this report's scope is enormous given the variety of interventions being considered. It would have not been feasible to systematically conduct updated searches for primary literature for each of the interventions under consideration. We did, however, consider newer primary studies identified through expert input and resources like the AoA compendium when applicable and we discuss them if they added to the body of literature already cited.

Non-pharmacological Interventions for Behavioral Symptoms of Dementia

Reviewer	Comment	Response
Are there any studies on non-pharmacological interventions for behavioral symptoms of dementia that we have overlooked?		
1	Yes. Missing studies on the following types of interventions that were to be included in this review: • Psychotherapy (e.g., behavioral management techniques; cognitive rehabilitation; cognitive stimulation therapy; reality orientation) • Smart home technologies	The initial review of psychotherapeutic techniques incorrectly ruled out behavior management techniques as being administered by the caregiver and therefore included in a separate ESP report. In light of the feedback, we re-examined the literature on behavior management techniques and include this as a section in the updated report. The report included smart home technologies such as tracking devices, motion detection devices, and home alarms within the section on wandering. No additional reviews meeting our quality criteria reviewed research on smart home technologies targeting symptoms other than wandering.
2	Yes. Among the interventions that were to be focus of review were "psychotherapy (e.g., behavioral management techniques…") They are notably absent in the report. My review of this literature indicates that there are a number of well-done studies that have demonstrated the utility of behavioral management approaches to decrease dementia-related behavioral problems. I'd like to bring one leading article to your attention: Logsdon, R.G., McCurry, S.M., & Teri, L. (2007). Evidenced-based psychological treatments for disruptive behavior in individuals with dementia. Psychology and Aging, 22, 28-36. The authors utilize the American Psychological Association's criteria for identifying evidence based treatment to review studies in this area. They conclude (from the abstract): "Results of this review indicate that behavioral problem-solving therapies that identify and modify antecedents and consequences of problem behaviors and increase pleasant events and individualized interventions based on progressively lowered stress threshold models that include problem solving and environmental modifications meet EBT criteria." The specific studies that they identify as meeting EBT criteria are delineated in the article.	The initial review of psychotherapeutic techniques incorrectly ruled out behavior management techniques as being administered by the caregiver and, therefore, was included in a separate ESP report. In light of the feedback, we re-examined the literature on behavior management techniques and include this as a section in the updated report. We have included the Logsdon et al. (2007) article in the updated report.
2	Other review articles worth mention include: Allen-Burge, R., Stevens, A.B.,& Burgio, L.D. (1999). Effective behavioral interventions for decreasing dementia-related challenging behavior in nursing homes. International Journal of Geriatric Psychiatry, 14, 213-232. Kasl-Godley, J. & Gatz, M. (2000). Psychosocial interventions for individuals with dementia: An integration of theory, therapy, and a clinical understanding of dementia. Clinical Psychology Review, 20, 755-782. Cohen-Mansfield, J. (2001). Nonpharmacological interventions for inappropriate behaviors in dementia: A review, summary, and critique. American Journal of Geriatric Psychiatry, 9, 361-381.	We reviewed all of these articles, and none met our quality criteria for inclusion in the report. Additionally, similar articles which met our quality criteria are included in the report and adequately cover the topics in these suggested articles (Ayalon et al., 2006; Livingston et al., 2005; & Logsdon et al., 2007).

Non-pharmacological Interventions for Behavioral Symptoms of Dementia

Reviewer	Comment	Response
2	Also, in one of the review articles cited in your report, the authors draw favorable conclusions about the utility of behavioral interventions for dementia. Livingston et al. (2005). Systematic review of psychological approaches to the management of neuropsychiatric symptoms of dementia. American Journal of Psychiatry, 162, 1996-2021. "Only behavior management therapies, specific types of caregiver and residential care staff education, and possibly cognitive stimulation appear to have lasting effectiveness for the management of dementia-associated neuropsychiatric symptoms…" (from the abstract)	Noted. See response to previous comments re: inclusion of behavior management techniques as a section in the updated report.
3	No. The analysis was very carefully done.	Noted.
1	If you have not already, I suggest you also look at the following compendium from Administration on Aging (AoA). This was also used by the Portland ESP group that did the recent report on Interventions for Non-professional Caregivers of Individuals with Dementia. • Administration on Aging's Alzheimer's Disease Supportive Services Program. Annotated Bibliography: Evidence-based interventions that target people with ADRD or their caregivers. 2010. http://www.aoa.gov/AoARoot/AoA_Programs/HCLTC/Alz_Grants/docs/EB2010.pdf	We reviewed the AoA compendium for relevant, recent studies related to behavior management techniques and did not find any that met our criteria. Relevant studies included work by Linda Teri that was already included in the report, as well as other articles referencing behavior management techniques that were limited to assessing caregiver outcomes rather than patient outcomes.
4	Yes: Did not see relevant research by Burgio and Cohen-Mansfield (e.g., Burgio et al. 2002; Cohen-Mansfield et al., 2007), which provide further support for non-pharmacological approaches to managing dementia-related behaviors. Were these bodies of work included in the reviewed research?	Based on this feedback, we reviewed both primary articles. The Cohen-Mansfield article was included in the section on agitation as it was part of the Kong (2009) review that was cited in that section; we did not examine primary articles in this section of the report. Though the Burgio (2002) article was *cited* in the reviews included in the BMT section of our paper, it was not included as evidence in these reviews for the same reason that it is not applicable to this review. This research examines two BMT interventions with different staff training strategies. Because there is no control group receiving a non-BMT intervention, there is no way to examine the effects of BMT overall (only the relative efficacy of different types of BMT); therefore, any change in outcome could be due to maturation rather than intervention. Related work by Burgio was also included in the reviews cited in our report and, therefore, this research is represented in our overall reporting of results. Though these articles both provide some support for the effectiveness of certain behavior management techniques, unfortunately, neither one is methodologically rigorous enough to change our overall interpretation of findings.
5	The following study may be of interest. Wall M, Duffy A. The effects of music therapy for older people with dementia Br J Nurs. 2010 Jan 28-Feb 10;19(2):108-13.	This study was not included in the report because it was outside our search timeframe. In reviewing the findings, however, we noted that the authors of this paper came to the same conclusions as we did regarding the effectiveness of music therapy: Though initial research documents positive results in terms of reducing agitation, methodologically sound studies are needed to adequately support positive results.

Non-pharmacological Interventions for Behavioral Symptoms of Dementia

Reviewer	Comment	Response
Additional comments		
1	Executive Summary, Results • Key Question 1 (thru page ix) – o Missing information on several groups of interventions that were to be included in the review § psychotherapy – e.g., behavior management, cognitive rehabilitation, cognitive stimulation, reality orientation; § smart home technologies o Is there any summary statement on comparison of non-pharm interventions with each other, and with pharmacological approaches?	Noted. See response to previous comments re: inclusion of behavior management techniques as a section in the updated report. We added a summary statement on the lack of comparison information. See response to previous comment re: smart home technologies being covered in the section of the report on wandering.
1	• Key Question 2 (page ix) – o Missing information on several groups of interventions that were to be included in the review § psychotherapy – e.g., behavior management, cognitive rehabilitation, cognitive stimulation, reality orientation; § smart home technologies o Is there any summary statement on comparison of non-pharm interventions with each other, and with pharmacological approaches?	Noted. See response to previous comments re: inclusion of behavior management techniques as a section in the updated report. We added a summary statement on the lack of comparison information. See response to previous comment re: smart home technologies being covered in the section of the report on wandering.
1	Methods, Interventions (page 2) – Throughout the report • Missing information on several groups of interventions that were to be included in the review o psychotherapy – e.g., behavior management, cognitive rehabilitation, cognitive stimulation, reality orientation; o smart home technologies	Noted. See response to previous comments re: inclusion of behavior management techniques as a section in the updated report. See response to previous comment re: smart home technologies being covered in the section of the report on wandering.
1	Results, Wandering (page 28, 34, elsewhere?) – • Should add a reviewer who has a focus on wandering.	Done.
1	Results, Key Question 2 (page 33) • At end of this section, consider adding a statement about the comparison of non-pharm interventions with each other, and with pharmacological approaches. If there are no relevant studies, you could have a statement to that effect as you do on page 31 for Key Question 1.	Agreed. This statement has been added.
1	NOTE: Additional comments/suggested edits are shown in Track Changes on the document attached (mostly punctuation/grammar changes for clarification).	All edits included in the document were addressed. Because they primarily consisted of word grammar edits and are not in need of additional discussion, they are not itemized here.
2	I'd suggest adding behavioral interventions to one of the key areas addressed in this report.	Noted. See response to previous comments re: inclusion of behavior management techniques as a section in the updated report.
6	Page v, line 3: "We obtained additional articles from reference lists of pertinent studies." This method should be more fully explained below in "Study Selection and Quality Assessment"	Manual searching for articles that were not identified through the systematic search of electronic databases is a standard, supplemental search method used in conducting systematic reviews.

Non-pharmacological Interventions for Behavioral Symptoms of Dementia

Reviewer	Comment	Response
6	Page v, line 29: "cycles that individuals with dementia experience." Awkward?; Better: "cycles experienced by individuals with dementia?"	Agreed. This sentence has been changed.
6	Page x, line 1: "None of the systematic reviews captured in our search identified any head-to-head trials that directly compared safety among different non-pharmacological interventions, or between non-pharmacological and pharmacological treatments." Repeat of above text	This section of text refers to safety, while the previous text refers to effectiveness.
6	page 2, line 15: BY 'BEHAVIORAL MANAGEMENT TECHNIQUES DO YOU MEAN BEHAVIOR MODIFICATION ?: Behavior modification is the use of empirically demonstrated behavior change techniques to improve behavior, such as altering an individual's behaviors and reactions to stimuli through positive and negative reinforcement of adaptive behavior and/or the reduction of maladaptive behavior through its extinction, punishment and/or therapy.	Due to the broad range of interventions covered, as well as the need to group them into an accessible organizational framework, we chose to use the term "Behavior management techniques" to represent the variety of techniques which were investigated. We agree that many different terms are used in the field, though this choice of terminology is consistent with other articles (e.g., Logsdon et al., 2007, refer to "behavior management interventions and Livingston et al., 2005, refer to "behavioral management techniques").
6	Page 4, line 12: "We organized the literature into the following categories." Should you better explain the rationale underpinning your categorization schema? For example, couldn't ALL of listed categories be considered "Behavioral Management?"	All categories focus on reducing behavioral symptoms of dementia; however, we organized the review in a manner such that similar types of interventions were grouped, consistent with existing literature (e.g., Livingston et al., 2005). We agree that other organizational frameworks could have been considered, though we believe that this is the most parsimonious manner in which to adequately capture all relevant techniques.
6	Page 8, line 13: "With the exception of one small trial (N=17) that showed a benefit on mood," Needs citation?	We chose not to include citations because this text is in the summary of findings for this section. Citations are provided in the subsequent section that provides the results in greater detail.
6	page 10, line 7: "The review identified three additional studies that could not be combined in the meta-analysis; of these, two studies found that SPT was effective in reducing challenging behaviors, and the third found no overall benefit, and that the response to SPT may differ among individuals." Each and every study discussed in this work should be cited.	Because our overview of non-pharmacological interventions summarizes the work done previously by other systematic reviews, we refer to the systematic reviews themselves rather than the individual studies these reviews included. BMT was an exception to this format because we focused on the individual studies that had been identified by previous systematic reviews.
6	Page 18 line 7: "during the four week treatment period" May need hyphen.	This change has been made.
6	Page 19 line 27: Wide indeed! You may need to break this broad category into sub-categories? For example, functional behavior analysis, token economies and individualized behavioral reinforcement strategies are clearly categorizable as "Behavior Modification;" other inclusions here a "stretch…"	We considered many different ways of organizing this category. The reviews and even the individual studies included such a variety of intervention components that separating "specific ingredients" into subgroups was not possible. As noted above, due to the broad range of interventions covered, as well as the need to group them into an accessible organizational framework, we chose to use the term "behavior management techniques" to represent the variety of techniques which were investigated. We agree that many different terms are used in the field, though this choice of terminology is consistent with other articles (e.g., Logsdon et al., 2007, refer to "behavior management interventions and Livingston et al., 2005, refer to "behavioral management techniques").

Reviewer	Comment	Response
6	Page 20 line 2: "Three good quality systematic reviews, including a total of 31 studies, examined the effectiveness of behavior management techniques for the treatment of behavioral symptoms of dementia." Cite!	We agree and have added the citations to these 3 systematic reviews.
6	Tables 1 and 2. Table more effective/useful if column added to list primary author and date	Due to space limitations, we chose not to include the primary author list and, rather, included this information as citations within the table.
6	Page 35, line 21: MSS - need to define abbreviation.	This change has been made.
6	Page 42 line 30: "That cognitively impaired elderly adults are at increased risk of falls represents simultaneously a potential rationale for and risk of exercise programs." Should be cited!	The previous sentence documents this same point and includes 2 relevant citations.
6	References, page 53: Note font variation in ref #4	This change has been made.
1	I had some of the same thoughts about whether you can make any statement about relative efficacy or safety of non-pharm versus pharm approaches, even though there aren't head-to-head comparisons. Otherwise, the serious risks of pharmacological approaches gets lost….	We agree that, given the dearth of direct comparisons, statements implying a comparison of approaches are not warranted; therefore, we only included statements about the dearth of research rather than any statements about the relative efficacy and safety without adequate documentation of comparisons.
1	**Feedback on the new text on behavioral management techniques (BMT) found on pages 19-25, as well as pages vii, xi, 39, 43, 46, and 50:**	
1	1. Page 21, Table 1	
1	a. Is there room to add information on the study setting? (Table 2 has a column for Setting)	Due to the other information included in the table, there was no additional room for more study details, and we tried to include the most relevant information in the table.
1	b. Can you add a glossary of tests included in the "Outcomes" column, to spell out the abbreviations?	Yes. This has been added.
1	2. Page 23	
1	a. On this page and throughout the document – be consistent in use of present or past tense when giving study results (e.g., page 23, line 5 has past tense, "…Gitlin…was the only study…"; line 22 has present tense, "Though they use a more conservative p value…."	This change has been made.
1	b. Line 20 – define "Type 1 error"	This term has been defined.
1	c. Line 23 – define "p value"	This term has been defined.
1	3. Page 24	
1	a. Line 26 – Text says setting of the Teri, Huda, et al. (2005) study was nursing home, but title of the article in References section page 55, line 4 says assisted living staff. Please clarify setting of the study.	This correction has been made.
1	b. Line 26 – Not sure this is a comment for the report, but just to let you know – VACO Mental Health is currently pilot-testing an adaptation of the Teri STAR program in VA Community Living Centers.	Thank you for this information.
1	4. Page 25	

Reviewer	Comment	Response
1	a. Line 13 – says "…this report examined a broader range of primary studies…" – Does this sentence include the studies mentioned in the preceding bullets, or is this sentence referring to some other studies? (Maybe I just didn't follow correctly.)	This paragraph has been re-worded for clarity.
1	b. Line 22 – Define "grade of B"	We chose not to include additional information on this definition in text but provided additional contextual information in the report (i.e., describing the findings) so that readers could more easily interpret the grade-related findings. We have added a citation to the Oxford Centre for Evidence Based Medicine (http://www.cebm.net) for further information on their particular grading system.
1	**Feedback on other parts of the report:**	
1	1. General – Whenever possible, be consistent in order of results for the types of interventions – use same order in Executive Summary, Table of Contents, and in body of document.	We have examined the report for consistency in ordering of interventions and have made changes as needed to maintain consistency throughout.
1	2. Page vii, first paragraph, on TENS – Can you clarify the last sentence -- If no significant effects found in 3 RCTs, why say there is insufficient evidence? (e.g., poor quality studies, even though there were 3 RCTs?)	In order to clarify the conclusions, we have stated the conclusions made directly by the authors of the Cochrane review on TENS.
1	3. Page ix, Key Question 2 – If possible, use same order as in Key Question 1 summary of findings starting on page iv (put Behavior management techniques paragraph before Animal-assisted therapy….)?	This change has been made.
1	4. Page xiii, Appendix G, Reviewer comments – Just a reminder that these should be anonymous.	Noted.
1	5. Page 1, line 9 – "…placement of individuals with dementia into residential care."	This change has been made.
1	6. Page 3, line 4, "…home based care and ambulatory care; and extended care…." [remove comma after home-based care, and use semi-colon after ambulatory care?]	This change has been made.
1	7. Page 8 bottom, Page 9 top – Why not cite the individual studies and give their references (when possible), rather than the review references 10 and 11?	Because our overview of non-pharmacological interventions summarizes the work done previously by other systematic reviews, we refer to the systematic reviews themselves rather than the individual studies these reviews included. BMT was an exception to this format because we focused on the individual studies that had been identified by previous systematic reviews.
1	8. Page 9:	
1	a. Line 9 "…on problem behaviors." [Add references]	Given the broad scope of this report, whenever possible we summarized the findings of existing systematic reviews. Because in most cases we did not review the individual studies ourselves, we chose to refer only to the systematic review as the primary source.
1	b. Line 25 – "…in some individuals."	This change has been made.
1	c. Line 30 – "…among persons with dementia."	This change has been made.
1	9. Page 10, lines 4-5 and 8-11 – give references?	Please see response to item "8a" above.
1	10. Page 11:	

Reviewer	Comment	Response
1	a. Line 6 – give reference?	Please see response to item "8a" above.
1	b. Line 9 – give reference?	Please see response to item "8a" above.
1	c. Line 12 - …usual care."	This change has been made.
1	c. Line 12 - And add reference?	Please see response to item "8a" above.
1	11. Page 13 – Line 22 and line 27 – give references?	Please see response to item "8a" above.
1	12. Page 14 – Line 23 and line 29 – give references?	Please see response to item "8a" above.
1	13. Page 15	
1	a. Line 2 – remove comma after "dementia"	This change has been made.
1	b. Line 3 – remove comma after "massage"	This change has been made.
1	c. Line 9 – "…in persons with dementia in the…"	This change has been made.
1	d. Line 17 – "…preserved in individuals with dementia…"	This change has been made.
1	17. Page 17, line 25 – "…in persons with dementia…"	This change has been made.
1	18. Page 18, Line 1, line 3, line 8, line 11, line 14 – add references.	Please see response to item "8a" above.
1	19. Page 19, Line 8, line 9, line 10 – add references.	Please see response to item "8a" above.
1	20. Page 26	
1	a. Line 9 – Please clarify, is it the British National Institute for Health and Clinical Excellence?	Yes. This change has been made.
1	b. Lines 11-12 – Past or present tense (be consistent)	This change has been made.
1	21. Page 29, Table top row, column on Intervention - viewed (past tense)	This change has been made.
1	22. Page 30, Table second row, column on Setting – What kind of "Veterans home" – State Veterans Home?	The primary article describes the setting as a "20-bed special care Alzheimer's unit in a midwestern Veteran's home." The article provided no further details.
1	23. Page 33, line 24 – Spell out "BMI" if first time used.	This change has been made.
1	24. Page 35, line 21 – Spell out "MSS" if first time used.	This change has been made.
1	25. Page 36, line 21 – Do you mean, "…on the behavioral symptoms of agitation in dementia" here?	Yes. This has been edited for clarity.
1	26. Page 37	
1	a. Lines 21-23 – Says no systematic reviews on inappropriate sexual behavior. Did you check for individual studies on this topic?	Given the scope of this report, we did not search for individual studies on inappropriate sexual behavior. However, we recognize that it is an important topic that may warrant a focused systematic review of primary studies.
1	b. Lines 28-30 – Next sentence says the opposite of this sentence? (clarify?)	This has been clarified. There were no head to head studies; only one review attempted to examine results across studies by comparing effect sizes.
1	27. Page 38, line 8 – Can you add a concluding sentence for this paragraph?	This has been added.
1	28. Page 38, line 21 – Add reference number closer to name HTA to make clear it is ref 70.	This change has been made.
1	29. Page 40, line 7 – "The HTA report [add ref number here]…"	This change has been made.

Reviewer	Comment	Response
1	30. Page 59, bottom of first table on the page – "The symptoms, comparators, [add comma], outcomes and settings are best dealt with using inclusion and exclusion criteria; [use semicolon here]…"	This change has been made.
4	I am pleased to see this review of non-pharmacological approaches to managing dementia-related challenging behaviors. This is an area of important focus for VHA, especially in light of the lack of evidence for and increased death risk associated with the use of antipsychotics with older patients. The manuscript is generally comprehensive; below are some comments to consider as the report is finalized, in addition to the comments provided above.	Thank you for this feedback.
4	P. iii: "terms" is misspelled	This correction has been made.
4	Pp. iv-v: Behavior management interventions is referenced, but is not defined as other interventions are.	This section has been updated to include a definition.
4	At times the paper refers to "behavior management techniques" and at other times "behavioral management techniques". This should be made consistent.	This term is now consistently "behavior management techniques" throughout the report.
4	Behavior therapy is referred to throughout the report, though it is not clear what this specifically refers to.	While behavior management techniques are referred to throughout the report, behavior therapy is referred to only in relation to the agitation findings. This is the term used in the review cited within the agitation section. Due to space limitations, none of the interventions in this section (social contact, environmental modification, caregiver training, and behavior therapy) were defined, under the assumption that readers could examine the cited systematic review if they want more specific information than this included in this report.
4	P. 24: The summary of the Logsdon, Teri, et al.(1997) study states "yet there was no change on measures of cognition". Unless the reference to "cognition" is meant to refer to behaviors, this statement is unclear as one would not expect to see change in cognition from a behavior management intervention.	The wording of this summary has been changed to clarify the results.
4	Aggregating the results of studies across different settings (and patient populations with presumably different levels of dementia and behavioral severity) may attenuate findings, especially perhaps in studies examining behavior management interventions. Recommend reporting results/conclusions separately for different settings, to the extent possible.	We considered many different organizational strategies, and reviewed existing literature for models (e.g., Livingston et al., 2005). The reviews and even the individual studies on behavior management techniques included such a variety of intervention components that separating "specific ingredients" into subgroups was not possible.
4	Similarly, studies on behavior management techniques are aggregated in the report. This category represents a very broad array of interventions, thus limiting its internal validity and potentially contributing unclear or inconsistent findings.	We agree that the broad range of interventions and intervention components limit our ability to draw conclusions from this body of literature. We did look at each study and individual interventions, but there was very limited data for any single study and individual interventions. Therefore, it's difficult to conclude that there is a strong body of evidence for any single intervention.

Non-pharmacological Interventions for Behavioral Symptoms of Dementia

Reviewer	Comment	Response
4	P. 36: It is stated that "there is no evidence demonstrating an effect of various of social contact, environmental modification, caregiver training, combination training, or behavior therapy on the behavioral symptoms of dementia." This is unclear, as elsewhere in the manuscript evidence in support of one or more of these types of interventions is provided. Furthermore, this section is labeled as addressing agitation, yet the statement above relates more broadly to "behavioral symptoms of dementia". Furthermore, it is not clear whether some of Cohen-Mansfield's seminal work in this area was excluded.	This paragraph has been re-worded for clarity. Now the paragraph specifically refers to behavioral symptom of agitation. The review examined in this section (Kong, 2009) did include relevant Cohen-Mansfield work on this topic (1986, 2001); however, Cohen-Mansfield's (2007) work was not included in the review because the review search dates only extended through 2004. Based on this reviewer feedback, we obtained this primary article and updated the report accordingly. Thank you for this suggestion.
4	Pp. 42-43: Given that the greatest evidence reported was for behavior management interventions, it would seem that this should be reported earlier in the Discussion.	The discussion section has been ordered to follow the presentation of interventions in the rest of the paper, per reviewer requests; however, much of the discussion is devoted to behavior management techniques as we agree that these intervention strategies included the greatest evidence.
4	P. 50: The rating of "Low" level (versus, for example "Medium") of evidence assigned to behavioral management interventions seems inconsistent with the findings of the research reported in this area. While findings are not consistent across all studies, multiple RCTs (and other research) has provided some moderate level of support for (some of) these interventions. Further, as noted above, this category aggregates a wide range of different types of interventions that may contribute to inconsistent findings.	The rating of "low" rather than "medium" was used in reference to behavior management techniques because of the methodological concerns that occurred across studies. Inadequate blinding of raters, providers, and participants is a major threat to the internal validity of the existing studies, particularly as most outcomes were assessed by self-report or caregiver report; it is very likely that, following participation in what one knows to be the treatment condition, a participant or caregiver would (possibly inadvertently) provide a more positive rating on outcome measures simply due to being aware of participation. In addition to blinding concerns across all but one study, the reviewed studies also suffered from other threats to validity including using control groups that were non-intervention or waitlist controls, poorly defined/operationalized interventions, inadequately accounting for nesting, and inadequately adjusting for increased risk of a Type I error due to using multiple outcome measures. Though many of these studies reported positive results, the inconsistencies in results were noted both across studies and within studies. The inconsistent results included different results across timepoints as well as across measures assessing similar outcomes. We attempted to adequately describe the multiple positive findings reported by RCTs while also noting the methodological limitations across all studies. We agree that, overall, this area of research is promising; however, methodologically rigorous research conducted across research groups is needed to provide unequivocal support for the effectiveness of behavior management techniques.
2	Review of behavioral management techniques is a welcome addition to the report. Despite the many caveats raised in the report about the quality of studies of interventions for behavioral symptoms of dementia, behavioral management techniques appear to be some of the more promising interventions among them.	Noted. We agree and attempted to present the findings in such a way that this was presented in the BMT section and discussion.

Reviewer	Comment	Response
2	Comparison of non-pharmacological vs. pharmacological approaches regarding their relative safety (Key Question 2) and cost (Key Question 3).	
2	The report only draws conclusions when there are head-to-comparisons between non-pharmacological and pharmacological studies. Might it be possible draw some conclusions about these questions based on the broader aggregate of findings?	Because there was no research-based evidence on this topic, we chose not to include this information in the body of the report. This is because the strength of evidence is compromised when the effectiveness of two interventions is indirectly compared. However, we included this point in the discussion section of the report as we agree that this is an important consideration for future research directions.
2	On p. 1 of the report it notes: "Psychotropic medications are commonly used to reduce the frequency and severity of the behavioral symptoms of dementia. There is little evidence, however, that such interventions are effective, and their potential side effects are frequent and often hazardous. It has been reported that the use of atypical and typical antipsychotic medication is associated with the increased risk of death." In view of this, would it not be imprudent for the report to conclude that despite the mixed evidence for non-pharmacological interventions, they should be first line of treatment rather than pharmacological approaches? That is because non-pharmacological approaches are safe (vs. potentially serious side effects of medications) and some of them might be effective with certain behavioral symptoms or constellation of symptoms.	This is an important point to include in the discussion section, and we have included such a discussion in the report. We chose to include this in the discussion section rather than the body of the report because there is no research-based evidence to document on this topic.
2	Table 1, p. 21 I wasn't clear what the term "clustering" refers to.	The term "nesting" has been added to this table to clarify the meaning of the column header.
2	P. 36, lines 19-22: "Overall, there is no evidence demonstrating an effect of social contact, environmental modification, caregiver training, combination therapy, or behavior therapy on the **behavioral symptoms of dementia**." Since this section discusses studies of agitation, shouldn't this read "...**on symptoms of agitation in dementia**."?	This paragraph has been edited for clarity.
5	Page iv, line 2—for what years were the primary studies searched?	The search for primary studies for animal-assisted therapy was conducted from database inception through 12/9/2009, as noted in Appendix B.
5	page iv: Results. I find this section confusing. "We identified 22 good quality systematic reviews in *single* nonpharmacological interventions plus 8 good quality reviews" (lines 8 and 9). The rest of this paragraph mentions 10 reports (line 10), 12 reports (line 11), 3 reports(line 12), 3 reports (line 14), 5 reports (line 15) and 1 report (line 16). These reports add to 34 reports.	Yes, some of the reports reviewed multiple interventions and are therefore included in more than one subsection; therefore, reports used in subsections are not additive due to the fact that they are not mutually exclusive. The number of reports was inconsistent with other areas of the report, however, and this inconsistency has been corrected.

67

Non-pharmacological Interventions for Behavioral Symptoms of Dementia

Reviewer	Comment	Response
5	Throughout the document, the terms "behavioral symptoms", "behavioral problems", and "behavioral disturbances" "seem to be used interchangeably. If these terms each mean something different, could definitions. For example: The three key questions all use the term "behavioral symptoms" but many of the discussions use "behavioral problems" and "behavioral disturbance." The Background section (page 1) uses both the terms "behavioral problems" and "behavioral symptoms". If the terms all refer to the same thing, would it be helpful to use only one term?	This terminology has been made consistent throughout the report; now, behavioral symptoms is referred to throughout the document.
5	Page 2, line 10. "Population is adults with mild, moderate, severe dementia." Since there are several types of dementia, did studies discriminate between types of dementia? How does this report define "dementia?"	We proposed to use broad categories of dementia in our scope and objectives, in order to not limit the population of interest. Our search strategy in Appendix A shows the various terms we used to search for dementia in the literature. We relied on the definitions and diagnostic criteria used by the individual systematic reviews and the primary studies they included.
5	Page 3, line 26: Categories of drugs are mentioned with the exception of memantine which is the only medication listed by name. To be consistent, might want to say NMDA receptor antagonist rather than memantine.	This change has been made.
5	Page 6, line 5 states that 28 systematic reviews were included—seems inconsistent with what is reported in Executive Summary.	This inconsistency has been corrected.
5	Figure 1, page 7 is confusing—I am not following how the numbers add up	Some of the reports reviewed multiple interventions and are therefore included in more than one subsection; therefore, reports used in subsections are not additive due to the fact that they are not mutually exclusive.
5	Page 9: Discussion on reminiscence therapy refers several times to "problem behaviors"—not sure what these problem behaviors are that were assessed in the systematic review on reminiscence.	This terminology has been made consistent throughout the report; now, behavioral symptoms is referred to throughout this section and the entire document.
5	The section on Behavior Management Techniques (page 19-20) does not have any citations although various reviews and studies are mentioned. This might pose a problem for readers wanting to obtain additional information about these techniques	We agree and have cited the systematic reviews.
5	The sections on cognitive/emotion-oriented interventions and sensory-stimulation interventions are straightforward. The Behavior Management Techniques section is less clear. The explanation of behavior management techniques (page 19, lines 27-31) is vague—what is meant by "functional analysis of specific behaviors"? What are "token economies". What is meant by habit training—what habits?	These terms have been clarified in the report.
5	Table 1 on pages 21 and 22 seem disconnected from the discussion on pages 23 and 24.	We chose to include the table in text to summarize the entire behavior management technique section.
5	The bullet points on page 24, describing specific study findings, do not correspond to the order in which the studies are mentioned in Table 1. A reader, reading the bullet points on page 24, may want additional information about a particular study. The reader then has to read the table to try and match the references. Would it be better to have the bullet points reflect the same order of the studies in the table.	The table and bulleted list are in the same order.

Reviewer	Comment	Response
5	Page 25, line 13: "Though the three reviews cited in this report . . . " Not clear which "3 reviews" are being discussed here—there are more than three reviews discussed in this report.	This sentence has been clarified.
5	I am not clear why Table 1 and Table 2 are embedded in report but there are no tables embedded for sections on cognitive/emotion-oriented interventions, sensory-stimulation interventions, wandering, or agitation.	These were the only two sections which included primary studies and therefore we included evidence tables for only these two sections in the report.
5	There seems to be some inconsistency as to what the interventions are called throughout the report—sometimes they are "therapies", sometimes "treatments", sometimes "non-pharmacological interventions", sometimes "psychosocial therapies", and sometimes "approaches".	These terms are used interchangeably throughout the report; specifically, we tried to use terminology reflective of the terminology used in the various reviews we were citing and, therefore, we used all of these terms in the report.
5	Conclusion section is good.	Noted.
5	Page 42, line 21 mentions that masters level personnel are required for the emotion-oriented approaches. The only other place in the report that level of education for the interventionist is mentioned is in Table 1. If level of education is relevant (and I think it is), perhaps education should be mentioned in the text of the report when discussing emotion-oriented approaches.	We have added additional information to other sections of the discussion; additionally, information on degree requirements is included in Table 3.
5	As a clinician reading the conclusion, I might be interested in and want to read more about a particular intervention that shows some promise. I think it would be helpful to include the citations when discussing these interventions. For instance on page 43, line 4, it would be helpful to provide the citation for those studies that "suggest that behavior management techniques are effective strategies to reduce behavioral symptoms of dementia."	We have included a reference to Table 1 in this section of the discussion.